ARTHRITIS

**Questions
you
have
. . . Answers
you
need**

Other Books From The People's Medical Society

Take This Book to the Hospital With You

How to Evaluate and Select a Nursing Home

Medicine on Trial

Medicare Made Easy

Your Medical Rights

Getting the Most for Your Medical Dollar

Take This Book to the Gynecologist With You

Take This Book to the Obstetrician With You

Healthy Body Book: Test Yourself for Maximum Health

Blood Pressure: Questions You Have . . . Answers You Need

Your Heart: Questions You Have . . . Answers You Need

The Consumer's Guide to Medical Lingo

150 Ways to Be a Savvy Medical Consumer

Take This Book to the Pediatrician With You

100 Ways to Live to 100

Dial 800 for Health

Your Complete Medical Record

Diabetes: Questions You Have . . . Answers You Need

ARTHRITIS

Questions
you
have
... Answers
you
need

By Ellen Moyer

≡People's Medical Society®

Allentown, Pennsylvania

The People's Medical Society is a nonprofit consumer health organization dedicated to the principles of better, more responsive and less expensive medical care. Organized in 1983, the People's Medical Society puts previously unavailable medical information into the hands of consumers so that they can make informed decisions about their own health care.

Membership in the People's Medical Society is $20 a year and includes a subscription to the *People's Medical Society Newsletter.* For information, write to the People's Medical Society, 462 Walnut Street, Allentown, PA 18102, or call 610-770-1670.

This and other People's Medical Society publications are available for quantity purchase at discount. Contact the People's Medical Society for details.

ISBN 1-882606-01-9

5 6 7 8 9 0
First printing, April 1993

CONTENTS

INTRODUCTION

More than 36 million Americans suffer from arthritis—a disease blind to economic or social status. While generally thought of as a disease of aging, various forms of arthritis can strike even the very young. Even its manifestations can differ among the people who have it: For some people it is a mild inconvenience. For others it is a debilitating crippler.

The bad news is that arthritis has no cure. Nor is there a surefire way to prevent it from occurring.

But the good news is that there are many effective and proven treatments that help relieve the suffering.

Each year millions of Americans spend billions of dollars seeking relief from the pain and the sometimes devastating effects of arthritis. Some of the money is well spent, and some completely wasted.

Because there is no cure, arthritis treatment is often associated with medical hucksterism. Remedies that have no record of effectiveness are sold to or thrust upon unsuspecting people, often by persons with no training whatsoever and sometimes even by highly educated medical professionals.

That is why we have written *Arthritis: Questions You Have . . . Answers You Need.* It is essential for anyone who has arthritis to fully understand her condition and to learn who treats it, what treatments work and where to turn when more help is needed.

As the nation's largest consumer-health advocacy organization, the People's Medical Society is dedicated to getting helpful and healthful information to the consumer. It is our philosophy that an informed consumer is an empowered one—a person capable of making the best health-care decisions in partnership with her health provider.

Utilizing a question-and-answer format, *Arthritis: Questions You Have . . . Answers You Need* is a compilation of the most often asked questions and the latest research from the medical literature about matters related to arthritis.

So while there is no cure for arthritis, the information you'll find in the following pages will help ease the pain.

Charles B. Inlander

Charles B. Inlander
President
People's Medical Society

Terms printed in boldface can be found in the glossary, beginning on page 173. Only the first mention of the word in the text will be boldfaced.

We have tried to use male and female pronouns in an egalitarian manner throughout the book. Any imbalance in usage has been in the interest of readability.

1 WHAT'S GOING ON INSIDE THIS JOINT?

Q: Let's start at the very beginning.
What exactly is arthritis?

A: *Arthro* is the Greek word for joint, and *-itis* means
inflammation. So, simply, arthritis is **inflammation**
of a joint, or several joints. Some forms of arthritis inflame
more than just joints, however, and at least one form of
arthritis, **osteoarthritis**, may cause very little inflammation.

Q: What exactly is osteoarthritis? And what other
kinds of arthritis are common?

A: Briefly, because we'll go into this in more detail soon,
osteoarthritis is kind of a "wear-and-tear" arthritis,
usually caused by joint injuries or old age, and is the most
common type of arthritis.

Both **rheumatoid arthritis** and **gout** are also fairly
common. Rheumatoid arthritis involves joint inflammation
and frequently affects your whole body. Gout involves one
or a few inflamed joints, too. It occurs when **uric acid
crystals** form in a joint.

Q: Okay, maybe you should explain inflammation.
What is it?

A: Most of the time, inflammation is the body's protective response to an injury or infection. The classic
signs—heat, redness, swelling and pain—are produced as a
result of biochemicals secreted by your body's infection-
fighting immune cells as they attempt to wall off and destroy

germs and to break down and remove damaged tissue. Usually, once the battle is won, inflammation subsides.

Inflammation can also occur when, for reasons not clearly understood, the body's immune system turns renegade and attacks its own tissue. That seems be what happens with rheumatoid arthritis. Some researchers think it takes both a genetic tendency and exposure to a virus or other "bug" to initiate this immune-system change. But we're getting ahead of ourselves. Next question, please.

Q: So there is inflammation with rheumatoid arthritis and other **rheumatic diseases**, right?

A: Both **acute** (sudden and severe) and **chronic** (ongoing) inflammation are possible with rheumatoid arthritis and other rheumatic diseases. Osteoarthritis, on the other hand, may cause only mild inflammation or none at all.

Q: I know that joints include the knees, hips, knuckles and the like. But the truth is, that's about *all* I know. Are there other joints?

A: Any place in the body where two or more bones meet is considered a joint. Most, but not all, joints allow you to move, bend, even twist and turn to some extent. Some joints, such as those between the vertebrae in your back, are designed to be very strong and allow only slight movement. Others—your wrists, for instance, and the other joints in your arms and legs—are quite flexible.

There are hundreds of joints in the body. Besides letting you walk and talk, joints help you breathe. The joints connecting your ribs to your **sternum** and spine allow your chest to expand when you inhale. You'll find joints in your skull (saw-toothed suture joints that harden once your brain reaches its full size), your middle ear (where they allow a tiny bone to vibrate), even where the roots of your teeth are embedded in your jawbone.

Q: Can you develop arthritis in any joint?

A: Arthritis doesn't normally strike every joint, but there are a lot of places where it can settle. And different forms of arthritis tend to prefer different joints. Osteoarthritis seems to prefer hips, knees and hands, for instance, while gout—another form of arthritis—often zeroes in on your big toes. That's a very general look at the joints affected by arthritis; later we'll elaborate on the specific forms of arthritis and their manifestations.

By the way, doctors often use the term **articular** in reference to a joint. (In general, it means "the place of junction between two discrete objects.") Don't let some fancy term like *periarticular* throw you either. It simply means "around the joint." And the prefix *arthro-* or *arthr-* at the beginning of a word refers to a joint or joints.

Q: What holds a joint together? Muscles?

A: Muscles and **tendons** (which connect muscles to bone) play a mostly minor role in keeping joints stable. Actually, **ligaments**—strong, **fibrous** bands that connect bone to bone—wrap around joints like a nest of rubber bands and keep them stable.

Take the knee, for instance. It has four ligaments that are pretty well known, at least to football players, or even backyard athletes who land hard the wrong way. There is a collateral ligament on each side of the knee and two that cross over in the back. But six additional lesser-known ligaments also hold the knee together.

The structure of some bones helps hold joints together, too. For instance, both the hips and shoulders have a ball-and-socket design that allows these joints to rotate, usually without becoming dislocated.

Q: So what keeps the bones from grinding against each other like a mortar and pestle?

A: In a healthy joint, the ends of both bones are covered with a tough, rubbery, supersmooth tissue called **cartilage**. Cartilage allows the bones to glide past one another with little friction.

In addition to cartilage, each joint is encased in a tough, fibrous, fluid-filled **joint capsule**. The cells lining the inside of the capsule form the **synovial membrane**, or **synovium**. These cells perform a vital function. They secrete **synovial fluid**, which is to your joints what oil is to your car's engine. Synovial fluid provides protective lubrication to the joint and helps to nourish the cartilage. Synovial cells are seriously and permanently altered by rheumatoid arthritis.

Q: Short of dissecting the family hamster, is there any good way for me to see what a joint looks like?

A: The next best thing to seeing a live one is to consult a good anatomy book. We suggest *Anatomy of the Human Body* by Henry Gray (Philadelphia: Lea & Febiger, 1985), a classic of detailed drawings that's available in many college or hospital libraries.

To orient yourself right now, see the drawing of a typical knee joint below.

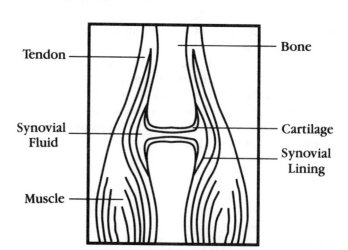

2 JOINTS GONE BAD

Q: You've briefly described three types of arthritis —osteoarthritis, rheumatoid arthritis and gout. But I don't really understand them. What are they? How are they different?

A: Osteoarthritis was once considered solely a "wear-and-tear" disorder. Now most doctors believe that it doesn't have a single cause and probably results from a combination of genetics and joint mechanics, such as mis-alignment. Osteoarthritis involves the breakdown of that slippery-smooth surface tissue—cartilage—in a joint, and is most often associated with old age and joint injuries. It never involves other parts of your body, but it can be painful.

Rheumatoid arthritis is a completely different disorder and the more serious of the two. It involves joint inflam-mation and breakdown, whole-body symptoms of fatigue, loss of appetite and weight loss, and sometimes inflammation in parts of the body besides the joints.

Gout is inflammation and swelling in one or a few joints— usually toes, but sometimes other joints, too. The inflam-mation is caused by the formation of tiny needle-shaped crystals in the synovial fluid. The crystals are the result of a buildup of uric acid in the fluid. Gout is often the result of too much of certain foods and wine, but it has other causes as well. It is easily treated with a drug, **colchicine**.

Q: Who should I turn to if I suspect I have any one of these diseases?

A: Even if you suspect one particular type or the other, it may be best to talk with your family doctor first, before you attempt a self-diagnosis. Your doctor may be able to diagnose and treat you, especially if you have only mild osteoarthritis. Or she may send you to a **rheumatologist**, a doctor who specializes in diagnosing and treating arthritis and other rheumatic diseases. We'll talk more about rheumatologists later, but we should mention now that arthritis patients say these specialists are usually very helpful.

Q: How does a doctor figure out whether I have arthritis?

A: Think of your doctor as a detective. Your joints hurt, and her job is to figure out why—in other words, to come up with an accurate diagnosis.

First, she has to determine if indeed you have arthritis by ruling out other possible conditions that could cause similar symptoms. Is it possible you could have a joint injury—torn cartilage, for instance—or a muscle or ligament injury? Or maybe you have some other type of inflammation, such as **bursitis** or **tendinitis**? A bone tumor? A fracture?

If it's none of the above, there's more of a chance that you actually do have arthritis. So the doctor's second job is to figure out what kind of arthritis you have. Initially, she needs to distinguish between osteoarthritis and some sort of rheumatoid disease, including rheumatoid arthritis.

If it seems that you have rheumatoid arthritis or some other sort of inflammatory arthritis, she'll next try to pinpoint the type. Is it gout? Rheumatoid arthritis? **Lyme disease**—an increasingly prevalent tick-transmitted form of arthritis? Or maybe even **fibromyalgia**, an achy-all-over condition that is frequently mistaken for Lyme disease these days?

In the early stages of arthritis, it's not always easy to tell just what's happening and what's causing your problem. One thing is important, though. Your doctor needs to make sure you don't have an infected joint—yes, yet another type of arthritis is **infectious arthritis**—because an infected joint needs to be treated promptly with antibiotics. And she should be sure you don't have Lyme disease, because that, too, needs to be treated promptly with antibiotics.

Q: How does my doctor do all this?

A: Your doctor should first ask you a lot of questions about your pain. Remember that your answers can provide valuable clues, so try to be as specific and detailed as possible. When did it start? What were you doing? Has the joint ever been injured? Does it hurt more when you move it a certain way or when you've been on it for a while? Does it seem to snap, crackle or pop when you move it? Does it hurt while you're resting? Is it swollen, red, stiff? Do you have other symptoms? Fatigue? Fever? Weight loss? Have you had any recent infection? Any mysterious rashes? Bowel problems? Do you have a family history of arthritis?

Q: What about a physical examination?

A: Your doctor will examine your joints. She'll feel around them with her fingers and move them or have you move them as far as you can. Since several diseases mimic rheumatoid arthritis in its early stages, your doctor may want to do a complete physical examination.

Based on your answers to her questions and her findings when she examines your body, your doctor will probably want to order some tests. Chances are pretty good she'll order some x-rays to look for joint damage. And she'll probably order some blood tests to find out if you do indeed have inflammation present somewhere in your body.

If your doctor thinks you have an infected joint or gout, she'll withdraw some fluid from that joint to examine for bacteria or for the uric acid crystals that cause gout. Your doctor might also order a blood test for Lyme disease.

We'll go into more detail on specific diagnostic tests later, but first—do you have any more questions concerning the different types of arthritis?

Q: It seems like there are many forms of arthritis. Is that true?

A: You bet. More than 100 conditions belong in the family of what doctors call rheumatic diseases, which involve inflammation and degeneration of **connective tissue** and related structures. They can affect the joints and other connective tissues in the body, including the muscles, tendons and ligaments, heart and lungs, skin and eyes, as well as the protective coverings of some internal organs.

The family tree of rheumatic diseases includes the types of arthritis we've already mentioned plus some others: gout, a form of arthritis partial to big toes; Lyme disease, a tick-transmitted form of arthritis; **systemic lupus erythematosus**, or simply, lupus, a chronic inflammation of tissues and organs; **scleroderma**, a condition that involves thickening of the skin and changes in blood vessels and the immune system; and others. Although many are potentially life threatening, most respond to medical treatment.

Q: Wow, that's a lot of diseases. How many people have arthritis?

A: Many, unfortunately. According to the National Institute of Arthritis, Musculoskeletal and Skin Disorders, more than 37 million Americans have some form of arthritis or a related disease. Approximately 2.1 million people have rheumatoid arthritis. And almost everyone over age 60—some 43 million people—has some form of osteoarthritis, although only about half of those people have symptoms of pain and stiffness.

Q: Do only old people get arthritis?

A: No. Although the incidence of osteoarthritis starts to increase steadily in people age 45 or older, rheumatoid arthritis tends to hit people between ages 35 and 50. Lupus usually affects women of childbearing age. Lyme disease can strike anyone. **Ankylosing spondylitis**, a condition that leads to stiffening of the spine, occurs most frequently in men ages 16 to 35. And, as its name implies, **juvenile rheumatoid arthritis** affects children.

Q: Who's more likely to get arthritis— women or men?

A: That depends on the type of arthritis. Women are three times more likely than men to develop rheumatoid arthritis and nine times more likely to develop lupus. They're also the primary victims of scleroderma. But men are three times more likely to develop ankylosing spondylitis, and they hold a virtual monopoly on gout.

Osteoarthritis is pretty much an equal-opportunity disease. Men are only slightly less likely to get it than women.

Q: Which joints is arthritis most likely to affect?

A: Again, that depends on the type of arthritis. Osteoarthritis can affect any joint, but it commonly occurs in the hips, knees, feet and spine. It can also affect some finger joints, the joint at the base of the thumb, and the joint at the base of the big toe. It rarely affects the wrists, elbows, shoulders, ankles or jaw, unless the joint has been injured.

Rheumatoid arthritis may first cause pain in your hands, wrists, feet or knees. It can also affect your elbows, shoulders, neck, hips and ankles and, less commonly, just about any other joint, including the jaw.

Gout has a well-known reputation for settling in the big toe, but it can also occur in the hands, wrists, knees, elbows or instep of the foot.

Ankylosing spondylitis affects the spine, usually starting around the **sacroiliac joints**—your "tailbone"—causing lower-back and hip pain and stiffness. It can also inflame and stiffen the fibrous cords that connect the ribs to the spine and to the breastbone, making it hard to take deep breaths. Also sometimes affected are the heels, making it uncomfortable to stand on hard surfaces.

Q: All this sounds painful, but does it get any worse? Does arthritis cripple people?

A: It can, but for most people it doesn't have to. With proper medical care, including joint replacement, and some lifestyle adjustments (walking instead of jogging, for instance, or using a low stool instead of kneeling), most people with arthritis can continue to work, play, reproduce and take care of themselves and their families, although they may have some difficulty and pain doing so.

Studies show that after 10 to 12 years with rheumatoid arthritis, less than 20 percent of its sufferers are free of disability or deformity. On a cheerier note: Of those who do develop such problems, studies show that very few are using wheelchairs or are unable to take care of themselves. Most function independently, even though they have some difficulty performing some daily tasks.

Q: I've heard about people who required artificial joint replacements, for hips or knees, in order to function normally. How many people have arthritis this bad?

A: There are no statistics to show what percentage of people with arthritis eventually require an artificial hip or knee joint, according to David T. Felson, M.D., M.P.H., a rheumatologist and epidemiologist and associate professor of medicine at the Boston University Arthritis Center. However, the Center for Health Statistics figures that about 130,000 people with arthritis receive artificial hips each year. An additional 130,000 receive artificial knees.

OSTEOARTHRITIS

Q: Can you tell me some more specifics about osteoarthritis?

A: As we said earlier, osteoarthritis is sometimes called wear-and-tear arthritis, or **degenerative joint disease**. It involves the breakdown of cartilage and other tissues in a joint.

Osteoarthritis, or OA, is considered a chronic disease, as are rheumatoid arthritis and most other rheumatic diseases.

Q: **Uh oh. Doesn't chronic mean you have it for a long time?**

A: Right. Chronic means "persisting over a long period of time." Doctors use the word to refer to a disease that tends to stick around, even though its symptoms may come and go. Medical treatments can help to alleviate the symptoms of a chronic disease, such as the pain and stiffness of rheumatoid arthritis, and may even slow its course, but they seldom cure the disease. In other words, available treatments usually do not permanently relieve symptoms or tackle the cause of the disease.

Q: **And what do you mean when you say that osteoarthritis is a wear-and-tear disease? Are you saying that if you use your joints too hard you end up with osteoarthritis?**

A: Well, no, it isn't that simple. Some people's joints are good for a lot more miles than other people's. Lifelong marathon runners, for instance, are no more likely to develop osteoarthritis than anyone else. (Of course, they may be special, because the group doesn't include all the people who stopped running because of joint pain or injuries.)

Doctors do know that injured joints are more likely to develop osteoarthritis than joints that have never been injured. They also know that people who are overweight are more likely to develop osteoarthritis in their weight-bearing joints (the knees, mostly), presumably because a heavy load damages these joints. And they know that some people develop osteoarthritis at an age earlier than average, and that's apparently due to a genetic problem that affects their body's ability to manufacture an important component of cartilage.

In fact, doctors are trying to get away from the wear-and-tear concept and are looking instead at osteoarthritis more as a metabolic problem—one where the body can no longer provide the necessary upkeep and maintenance on a joint.

Q: Who gets osteoarthritis?

A: As we said before, people with injured joints, of course, and people who are overweight may develop osteoarthritis, especially at a younger age. So may people with inherited joint deformities (such as bowlegs or a dislocated hip, which can create uneven wear on cartilage) or people whose bodies have trouble making cartilage.

But just about anyone who lives long enough can expect to have some osteoarthritis. It's one of the oldest and most common diseases known to humankind. And it even affects animals.

A study that analyzed the x-rays of women's joints—the study looked at these x-rays for signs of cartilage deterioration typical of osteoarthritis—found osteoarthritis in only 2 percent of women younger than 45 years. Between the ages of 45 and 64, however, the prevalence was 30 percent. And 68 percent of women older than 65 years showed signs on x-rays of osteoarthritis. An important fact to keep in mind out of all this is that, even though you may have osteoarthritis extensive enough for it to show up on an x-ray, you may not have symptoms.

Q: What about men?

A: Remember we said earlier that osteoarthritis is an equal-opportunity disease. Men are slightly less likely to develop this form of arthritis.

Q: But suppose a person does have symptoms. What are they?

A: Osteoarthritis can creep up on you over a period of many years. Many people have mild aching and soreness in their joints, especially when they move. And a few people develop nagging pain, even when they're resting.

The joints tend to hurt most after they've been overused or after long periods of inactivity. It's common to have to work out some stiffness in the morning or after a long period of sitting, by walking and special stretches called **range-of-motion exercises**, which we'll describe later.

In its early stages, osteoarthritis often affects joints on only one side of the body. Rheumatoid arthritis, on the other hand, is usually **symmetrical**—that is, it usually affects the same joint on both sides of the body. And unlike rheumatoid arthritis, osteoarthritis usually doesn't cause inflammation of a joint or a general feeling of sickness. Rheumatoid arthritis may cause inflammation, fatigue, weight loss and fever.

Symptoms can be different in different joints, too. In your knees, you may feel a grating or catching sensation. In your hips, you may feel pain around the groin or inner thigh. In your fingers, you're more likely to develop bony growths, called **bone spurs**, that make your joints look swollen, even though they're not. Osteoarthritis in your spine may sometimes cause weakness or numbness in your arms or legs.

The pain of osteoarthritis can be severe at times. But sometimes the pain is bad for a year or so, then it lessens, at least temporarily, as the bone ends polish and smooth off.

Q: I know osteoarthritis can affect any joint but that it is most likely to occur in the hips, knees, feet and spine. Are all the other joints in the body immune from attack?

A: No. Osteoarthritis can also affect some finger joints, the joint at the base of the thumb, and the joint at the base of the big toe. Rarely, and usually as a result of an injury, osteoarthritis affects the wrists, elbows, shoulders, ankles or jaw. Ballerinas get osteoarthritis in their ankles, prizefighters in their knuckles, and racehorses in their much-abused forelegs.

Q: So osteoarthritis can be painful—that much I know. But how exactly does osteoarthritis affect a joint to cause such pain?

A: There are several stages of osteoarthritis, and in all of them there can be pain. To begin, the smooth cartilage covering the ends of the bones softens and becomes pitted and frayed. The cartilage loses its elasticity and is easily damaged by overuse or injury. Then, with time, large sections of cartilage may be worn away completely. Without this rubbery, shock-absorbing material, the bones rub together. That really hurts!

As the cartilage breaks down, the joint may change shape. The bone ends thicken and form bone spurs, where the ligaments and capsule attach to the bone. Fluid-filled **cysts** may form in the bone near the joint. And bits of bone or cartilage that have broken loose may drift around in the joint space, causing pain.

Q: How does a doctor determine if you have osteoarthritis?

A: He'll ask you to describe your symptoms and also ask about any physical stress or injuries that may have led to your pain. And he'll examine your joints, pressing them with his fingers and asking you to bend and straighten them as far as you can without pain.

A doctor can usually diagnose osteoarthritis based on your medical history and a physical examination. If he has any doubt about the diagnosis, though, he'll want to do some tests. If you have severe pain in many joints, for instance, or one joint in particular, it's a good idea to make sure you don't have rheumatoid arthritis or some other form of arthritis, or an infection or injury.

Q: So what kinds of tests might my doctor want to do?

A: For starters, he may want to x-ray your joints to see if they show the kinds of bone, cartilage and tissue changes typical of osteoarthritis. As we said earlier, joint pain is not always a good measure of joint damage. It's possible to have little pain with moderate joint damage, and some people have a lot of pain with only slight joint damage. An x-ray can help establish the actual amount of joint damage.

If you have a particular joint that's painful, your doctor may want to draw fluid out of the joint to check for infection, inflammation or the tiny crystals that cause gout.

And if you have inflammation or swelling, he may want to do some blood tests, including those used to diagnose rheumatoid arthritis. Those tests may include a **complete blood count**, an **erythrocyte sedimentation rate** test, and a test for **rheumatoid factor**. Later we'll discuss these tests in detail.

Q: Besides dying young, is there any way to prevent osteoarthritis?

A: True, osteoarthritis may develop for no apparent reason other than old age, but yes, there are several things you can do to lower your risk of developing osteoarthritis, says Marc C. Hochberg, M.D., M.P.H., professor of medicine, epidemiology and preventive medicine at the University of Maryland School of Medicine.

• Maintain your ideal weight to protect your knees and hips.

• Wear a seatbelt and shoulder harness to keep your knees (not to mention other body parts) from smashing into the dashboard if you have an accident.

• Avoid sports with a high potential for injuries— football, for instance. If you're playing contact sports, wear appropriate protective gear, such as knee pads and elbow pads.

• Exercise regularly, but choose an activity that's appropriate for your body type and level of fitness. Don't run if you're seriously overweight or have bad knees, for instance, or don't skateboard if you have osteoporosis. In other words, use common sense.

• Learn how to do your job as safely as possible, or change jobs if you have a job that's hard on a particular part of your body. If you're a carpet layer, for instance, you may want to use a low stool rather than kneel on your knees all day long. If you're a farmer, you may need to automate or hire some extra hands to spare your hips. Compared with the general population, farmers have a higher-than-average incidence of osteoarthritis of the hips, according to Dr. Hochberg.

RHEUMATOID ARTHRITIS

Q: Okay, now I know something about osteoarthritis. What can you tell me about rheumatoid arthritis?

A: Rheumatoid arthritis (RA for short) is a chronic disease that causes inflamed joints and that can affect other parts of your body, too, including connective tissues and the tissues that surround organs, such as your heart and kidneys. (More on that later.) It affects women two to three times more often than men. It can develop at any age, but most often shows up between the ages of 35 and 50.

Q: How can my doctor diagnose rheumatoid arthritis?

A: Diagnosis is easy in people with well-established RA, because they have obvious pain and swelling in symmetrical joints.

Arriving at a certain diagnosis is trickier, however, in people in the early stages of rheumatoid arthritis, when symptoms may be very mild and present in only a few joints. Several inflammation-producing diseases have similar symptoms, and it's hard to differentiate between them and RA.

Just as she does for osteoarthritis, your doctor will ask you about your symptoms—when they began, which joints are involved, whether you have other symptoms (such as fatigue or fever) and whether you've had any recent infections. Then she'll examine your joints, checking them for swelling, redness, stiffness and pain. She'll probably also order some blood tests and perhaps some x-rays.

Q: Since a certain diagnosis is not always easy to pinpoint, what should my doctor do or look for at the outset?

A: In a nutshell, your doctor should make sure you don't have a kind of arthritis with symptoms similar to RA that needs to be treated much differently than does rheumatoid arthritis.

Infectious arthritis, for instance, which is caused by a bacterial infection in a joint, needs prompt treatment with antibiotics, not **anti-inflammatory drugs**. So does Lyme disease, an arthritic condition caused by the bite of the tiny deer tick. (As we said earlier, a completely unrelated condition, fibromyalgia, is sometimes mistakenly diagnosed as Lyme disease.)

Q: **So what tests should my doctor order to rule out infectious arthritis and Lyme disease?**

A: Infectious arthritis is diagnosed by examining fluid from the infected joint, and Lyme disease through a history of your symptoms and by a blood test.

Q: **Back to rheumatoid arthritis—how does it affect a joint?**

A: RA strikes the joint capsules of the more flexible joints—those in your arms, hands, legs and feet. It inflames the normally delicate synovial membrane lining the joint capsule, thus affecting its normal functioning. This membrane, you'll recall, secretes joint-lubricating synovial fluid.

In rheumatoid arthritis, the synovial membrane thickens, overgrows and becomes fibrous. It develops folds and becomes a harbor for many kinds of immune cells, which secrete biochemicals that damage the tissues of the joint. Eventually, without treatment, the proliferating synovium and the misguided immune cells can erode away cartilage and **subchondral bone** (bone directly beneath the cartilage) and even begin to destroy the joint capsule and the ligaments holding a joint together. This is called joint deformity, and permanent joint deformity can occur within a year or two after onset of rheumatoid arthritis. Although studies have yet to confirm it, many doctors treating arthritis believe that permanent joint deformity can be minimized by early aggressive treatment with certain types of **disease-remittive** drugs. We'll discuss this in chapter 3.

Q: What causes RA?

A: No one knows for sure, and there may be more than one specific cause. One popular theory is that rheumatoid arthritis is an **autoimmune disease**, a disorder in which the body turns against itself and begins destroying its own cells and tissue. In fact, there's good evidence to support this theory, including blood tests that show immune-system abnormalities in people with rheumatoid arthritis. Another bit of evidence is the fact that drugs that suppress the immune system improve RA symptoms.

Q: What makes the immune system go haywire?

A: Nobody knows for sure. Many researchers think the disease is due to infection, perhaps from one or more undefined viruses or some other microorganisms, that somehow permanently alter the cells in the joint so that the immune system attempts to destroy them. In fact, certain types of arthritis are known to be caused by viral or bacterial infections, two of which we've already mentioned—infectious arthritis and Lyme disease. But so far, no particular virus or bacteria has been implicated as the cause of rheumatoid arthritis.

Many researchers think it takes a combination of exposure to a virus or other microorganism in conjunction with a genetic tendency toward the disease to cause the immune-system changes typical of an autoimmune disease.

Q: What do you mean by a genetic tendency? You mean if my mother or father had it, I'll get it, too?

A: Not necessarily. But if either of your parents or a brother or sister has rheumatoid arthritis, you are three to five times more likely than the general population to develop it yourself.

Q: What if more than one person in my family has RA? Am I certain to get it, too?

A: No one knows how high your risk climbs if more than one family member has RA.

Q: Can I get tested to see if I carry a genetic tendency to develop rheumatoid arthritis?

A: You would not normally be checked for this genetic tendency unless you were in a research study looking specifically for this sort of thing. Doctors say it's an unusual request, but it may be possible to have your blood drawn and sent to the nearest major laboratory where genetic testing can be done. The test is called HLA, or human leukocyte antigen, typing. By the way, the same sort of test is done to make organ transplant matchups.

Keep in mind, though, that you can carry **genetic markers** —specific genes—that increase your risk for rheumatoid arthritis and never develop any symptoms of the disease. "There are so many other factors involved in getting the disease that, as a predictor, this test is not considered particularly useful," says Kenneth Sack, M.D., clinical director of rheumatology services at the University of California School of Medicine in San Francisco. He and other doctors point out, too, that there's nothing you can do to prevent rheumatoid arthritis. "You don't order a test unless you know what you're going to do with the results," Dr. Sack says. "In my opinion, all a positive test will accomplish, possibly, is to make you worry about the future."

Q: What exactly is a genetic marker?

A: It's a spot or spots (called gene sites) on your **chromosomes**, the genetic material passed on to you from your parents and found in every cell in your body. Certain genes sites determine your hair color, blood type and many other characteristics about you. Other sites indicate a tendency to develop certain kinds of diseases.

HLA typing provides information about a set of genes that influence immune-system function. It can determine if you have genes that may put you at higher-than-normal risk of developing rheumatoid arthritis and other diseases. The test zeros in on certain proteins, called **antigens**, that stick to the surfaces of your white blood cells. It analyzes what proteins you have and, based on that, determines what genetic markers you have.

Q: Let's say I decide to get this HLA typing test. What is the normal range of genetic markers?

A: There is no "normal range" in HLA typing. Instead, the test maps gene sites. Results might look something like "A2, A12, B4, B8, C2, C4." The genetic marker HLA-B8 has been associated with lupus, HLA-B27 with ankylosing spondylitis, and HLA-DR4 with rheumatoid arthritis. A rheumatologist or a doctor familiar with genetic testing can explain the results.

Among rheumatic diseases, genetic testing has proven most reliable so far in association with ankylosing spondylitis. The genetic marker HLA-B27 is found in nearly everyone with symptoms of that disease.

Q: Enough about the invisible-to-the-eye markers for RA. What are the more overt indications, the symptoms?

A: Rheumatoid arthritis is an extremely variable disease —one that can present itself in many ways and that can change and evolve over time. That's one reason it isn't always easy to diagnose in its early stages or to predict exactly what its course will be for any one person.

In about two-thirds of people, rheumatoid arthritis begins with fatigue, lack of appetite, generalized weakness and mild, intermittent muscle and bone stiffness and pain. These symptoms may persist for weeks or months and baffle both you and your doctor.

Specific symptoms—early-morning stiffness and swollen, painful, hot joints—usually appear gradually as several joints, especially those of the hands, wrists, knees and feet, become affected, usually on both sides of the body. "These symptoms usually come on over the course of weeks or months, but sometimes it can take years for RA to reach its full form, at which time there is no question about the diagnosis," Dr. Sack says. In about one-third of people, symptoms may be confined to one or a few joints for months or years. Then more and more joints develop symptoms.

Q: Don't some people develop rheumatoid arthritis much more quickly than that?

A: Yes. About 10 percent of people with RA take only a few days to develop rheumatoid arthritis in several joints, often along with fever, swollen lymph nodes and an enlarged spleen. "We don't know why some people develop RA so acutely," Dr. Hochberg says. People with rapid onset of symptoms don't seem to stand out as being different from people whose symptoms develop slowly. They're not older, or younger or more likely to be male or female, and they show genetic markers for RA with about the same frequency as people whose symptoms develop slowly.

Interestingly, most studies seem to indicate that these people usually do *better* in the long run at avoiding permanent joint deformities than people whose symptoms develop gradually over time, Dr. Hochberg says. "It may be that they come to medical attention sooner and are treated earlier, before they have the chance to develop joint deformities," he says.

Q: I know you said rheumatoid arthritis can be quite variable in its course, but can you give me some idea of what to expect from this disease?

A: Expect unpredictability, for sure. "There are multiple courses of the disease," according to Dr. Hochberg. The mildest version of RA is called monocyclic, or one-cycle, rheumatoid arthritis. And, as its name implies, it's a one-shot deal. "The person develops rheumatoid arthritis, is treated, gets well and never has symptoms again," explains

Dr. Hochberg. They have no residual joint deformities or pain. People with monocyclic RA generally have symptoms for no more than a year or two and sometimes for just a few months. "There are no good numbers on how many people get this sort of RA," Dr. Hochberg says.

At the opposite end of the spectrum is malignant RA. People with this kind of arthritis don't respond to treatment, even with the full arsenal of anti-arthritis drugs. They develop joint deformities, usually within a few years of onset of their disease, and end up needing reconstructive joint surgery. Fortunately, only about 5 percent of people with RA develop this severe type.

Somewhere in between are the vast majority of people with rheumatoid arthritis. Most have symptoms that come and go over many years. Some people's symptoms never seem to get worse. Others have increasingly severe and prolonged **flare-ups**, and start to develop joint deformities.

All these people in the middle, with the more common manifestations of RA, do respond to one kind of treatment or another, at least for a time. Their symptoms settle down, or go into **remission** for a time, then flare up, again and again.

Q: You've been using the words flare-up and remission. What's a flare-up?

A: A flare-up is a period of time when your disease, in the form of symptoms, is acting up. "You have more pain, more fatigue, more stiffness, more swelling," Dr. Sack explains. Blood tests may indicate inflammation.

Q: How long can a flare-up last?

A: A flare-up can go on for days, weeks or months. According to experts, there is no particular time frame.

Q: And a remission?

A: In a manner of speaking, remission is when your symptoms have gone into hiding. That means morning stiffness lasts no longer than 15 minutes, you have no unusual fatigue and no joint pain or swelling, and blood tests show reduced inflammation.

Remissions can last weeks, months or years, but they are seldom totally without pain, Dr. Sack says. "Usually we see a partial remission, a little pain, a little of this, a little of that, but basically the patient says he or she feels much better."

Remissions can occur in response to treatment, but they also can occur spontaneously, independent of any known cause, in people with rheumatoid arthritis who are receiving no medical treatment. "We know almost nothing about spontaneous remission," Dr. Hochberg says. "We don't know why it happens."

Most people with RA have partial remissions. About 5 to 10 percent of all people with RA go into remission each year, and may stay in remission for a year or so until their arthritis flares up again.

Q: Does rheumatoid arthritis ever just burn out?

A: As a matter of fact, there is a condition that's sometimes called "burned-out" arthritis, although some doctors prefer not to use this term. People with burned-out arthritis no longer have flare-ups, so their joints are no longer swollen. Their blood tests measuring inflammation are close to normal. And they tend not to have the fatigue associated with RA.

But they often do have joint pain and disability as a result of their years of having had RA. "Burned-out arthritis may occur 10 or 20 years after the initial onset of the disease," Dr. Hochberg explains. "It's a long-term remission."

Q: Isn't it true that some people get only a touch of rheumatoid arthritis?

A: Yes, but they seem to be a lucky minority. Some people have only mild flare-ups with long remissions and never have much joint damage. When their blood is tested, these people often do not carry genetic markers for rheumatoid arthritis, nor does their blood show signs of inflammation.

Q: Is there a test my doctor can do to tell if I have rheumatoid arthritis?

A: There's no one test to confirm that you absolutely and without a doubt have rheumatoid arthritis. So your doctor can attempt to pinpoint your diagnosis in a number of ways. He'll ask you about your symptoms and the history of your joint pain. He'll bend, probe and feel around your aching joints and anywhere else you hurt. He'll order a few laboratory tests, and he may also order x-rays or other imaging techniques.

Q: Sounds like a lot of blood testing is done. Is that true?

A: Well, yes, three blood tests are pretty much standard in the early stages of diagnosis in order to help your doctor get a better idea of what's going on in your body: a complete blood count, an erythrocyte sedimentation rate test, and a test for rheumatoid factor (a protein that signals the presence of inflammation). Furthermore, your doctor can order specific blood tests to check for other types of arthritis or rheumatic diseases, such as Lyme disease or lupus.

Q: What's a complete blood count?

A: To start, you should know the medical acronym for it—CBC—because more often than not that's what medical and lab personnel call it. This test measures a number of components of your blood, including the number and quality of red blood cells (**hematocrit** and **hemoglobin**); the number and type of white blood cells; and the number of platelets (sticky cells that help blood clot). The complete blood count is the most frequently ordered medical test, and it helps give your doctor an idea of your general health.

Q: How does it do that?

A: Let's say you have chronic inflammation, as do many people with RA. In this case the number of red blood cells is usually reduced.

If you have an infected joint, you may have increased numbers of certain types of white blood cells, which fight infection.

Q: Okay, let's go on to the next blood test you mentioned. What's a sedimentation rate test?

A: A "sed rate" test—as it's often called in the medical world—can give a doctor an idea of how much inflammation, if any, is present in your body, which is something he cannot determine merely by examining your joints. This test measures how fast red blood cells cling together, fall and settle to the bottom of a special, graduated test tube. The more inflammatory proteins present in the blood, the faster these cells clump together and sink. So the faster your sedimentation rate, the worse your rheumatoid arthritis may be.

Keep in mind, however, that a sedimentation rate test simply indicates inflammation. Although it may suggest it, this test cannot prove you have rheumatoid arthritis. That's because inflammation can be caused by other conditions besides RA; infections, cancer, even unruptured acute appendicitis can boost sedimentation rates.

Q: You also said that another lab test looks for rheumatoid factor. What is rheumatoid factor?

A: In simple terms, it's a protein in your blood that indicates your body's immune system is turning against you.

"The presence of rheumatoid factor indicates that your immune system is trying to get rid of what it considers to be damaged or unwanted **antibodies**," explains Terry Phillips, Ph.D., director of immunogenetics and immunochemistry and associate professor of medicine at George Washington University Medical Center, Washington, D.C.

Q: What's an antibody?

A: An antibody is a type of blood protein made by the body in response to a foreign substance. The purpose of the antibody is to bind to the foreign substance and eliminate it from the body. But in the case of RA, the body is trying to get rid of an antibody that helps to put the brakes on inflammation.

Q: So the presence of this rheumatoid factor definitely means I have rheumatoid arthritis, right?

A: Not necessarily. Although about two-thirds of people with rheumatoid arthritis have rheumatoid factor in their blood, a positive test does not necessarily nail down your diagnosis. That's because a number of conditions besides rheumatoid arthritis are associated with the presence of rheumatoid factor. These conditions include lupus, tuberculosis, cancer and viral infections. And about 5 percent of

all people have rheumatoid factor and no signs of rheumatoid arthritis or any other disease.

Q: So what good is this test?

A: While it's not useful as a screening test, a rheumatoid
factor test can be used to confirm a diagnosis in
people who have signs and symptoms of rheumatoid arthritis.
Also, it can help identify people who may have particularly
aggressive arthritis. The more rheumatoid factor found in a
person's blood, the more likely he is to have RA that affects
more than just his joints.

Q: Is the blood ever checked for other things, too?

A: Blood can also be checked for a number of other red
flags for inflammation, called *acute phase reactants*.
Doing this can give your doctor an idea of the extent of
disease activity and the likelihood of progressive joint
damage. High levels of these reactants in the blood may
make your doctor more likely to recommend early, aggressive drug treatment.

And once you start taking drugs for arthritis, your doctor
should monitor your blood for possible drug side effects. We
talk more about this in chapter 3.

Q: My doctor used a needle to draw some fluid out of my swollen joint. Why?

A: Examining the synovial fluid from a swollen joint is
helpful in diagnosing a number of conditions, including RA. Your doctor is more likely to do this if only one
joint is inflamed. (If only one joint is inflamed, you more
likely have a joint infection or gout, a kind of arthritis caused
by crystals that have formed in the joint capsule.) If you've
already been diagnosed with rheumatoid arthritis and have a

swollen and inflamed joint that isn't responding to treatment, your doctor may take fluid from that joint to see if
it's infected.

He'll examine the fluid right in his office and may also
send it for additional tests.

Q: What's he looking for?

A: Joint fluid is examined for its appearance. Normal
synovial fluid is a transparent amber color. If the fluid
is cloudy or opaque, you probably have inflammation or an
infection in the joint.

Joint fluid is also examined for its viscosity, or lubricating
qualities. Like oil, the molecules in synovial fluid tend to
stick together, providing lubrication. A drop of normal
synovial fluid, squeezed from a syringe, has a long, fine tail.
Synovial fluid from an inflamed or infected joint does not;
therefore, it's a poor lubricant.

Joint fluid is also examined for the number of blood cells
it contains. Red blood cells in the fluid may mean the joint
has been injured. A high number of white blood cells indicates inflammation or infection. **Glucose**, or sugar, levels are
checked, too, and can indicate inflammation or infection.

If it looks like you have an infection, your doctor should
Gram-stain and **culture** the fluid he withdraws from the
joint. Often helpful because it multiplies the number of
microorganisms, making identification easier, a culture is the
growth of bacteria or microorganisms on a special material
that provides the microorganism with food.

In a Gram-stain test, dyes are added to the infected synovial
fluid. Certain bacteria stain in certain ways, and this helps
the doctor determine exactly what microorganisms have
taken up residence in your aching joint.

Under a microscope with a special polarizing filter, your
doctor can check your synovial fluid for tiny crystals. If the
fluid contains long needle-shaped crystals, you have gout,
not rheumatoid arthritis.

Q: Would a doctor ever take a sample of synovial tissue to analyze?

A: He might, especially if you have one joint that is persistently swollen and he's having a hard time figuring out what the problem is, even using the tests we just mentioned. It's possible to get a bit of this tissue using a special hollow-core needle. The doctor carefully inserts the needle into your joint capsule, punching out a plug of tissue about the size of a grain of rice.

Q: You mentioned x-rays earlier. What do they show?

A: Early in the disease, x-rays of affected joints are usually not helpful in establishing a diagnosis. They show only what is apparent from physical examination— namely that you have soft-tissue swelling and excess fluid in the joint capsule. However, x-rays can be used to determine if you have bone cancer. (This is most likely to be done if you've previously had cancer.)

Some doctors take what they call baseline x-rays before they begin treatment. They save these x-rays to compare with those taken later on, perhaps every year or two. This helps them determine the extent of cartilage destruction and bone erosion produced by the disease. Such information can help you and your doctor make decisions regarding drug therapy or even surgery, including when it's time to consider joint replacement.

Q: What about those fancy, expensive imaging techniques, like MRI? Are they helpful?

A: In special situations, **magnetic resonance imaging (MRI)** can be helpful, but it's not often used to diagnose rheumatoid arthritis. It's more likely to be helpful if your doctor thinks you have a mechanical problem, such as a dislocation, a misalignment or a ligament or cartilage tear in one of your major joints—a knee, shoulder, hip or wrist. MRI is also very useful in helping a doctor visualize nerve or disk problems in the spine, which sometimes occur with osteo-arthritis or ankylosing spondylitis.

Q: Are other imaging techniques ever helpful?

A: They can be. **Computerized axial tomographic scans**—CT or CAT scans, for short—can be very helpful troubleshooting problems in the spine, hips, pelvis and shoulders. The benefit of this technology in this case is that a CT scan provides you with a 3-D image of your bones.

Scans that use radioactive dyes also can provide important information about cell activity within your bones. These scans can detect cells that are rapidly dividing and growing, as they might with cancer, or that are dying off, as they do in some serious bone disorders. The latter condition is called **osteonecrosis**.

Q: So is that about it for the modern technology available to diagnose rheumatoid arthritis?

A: No, there's more. **Ultrasound**, a technique that uses high-speed sound waves to create images of internal organs, is sometimes used to assess joints. The sound waves bounce back when they hit solid objects, but go through fluids and air. The sound waves are transmitted from the tip of a device called a **transducer**, which is moved back and forth over the area to be imaged. Also in the tip is a sensitive microphone, which picks up the rebounding sound waves and transmits them to either an **oscilloscope**, an instrument that resembles a television screen, or to a receiver that records them permanently on paper.

Ultrasound can be useful in the detection of soft-tissue abnormalities around a joint that are hard to detect simply by feeling and bending the joint and that may not appear on an x-ray. For instance, **rheumatoid nodules** and cysts are best assessed by ultrasound. So are tendon injuries.

Q: **Seems like a lot of tests are available. How do I know if a test is necessary or useful for me? Or must I undergo them all?**

A: Before you agree to any test or procedure, find out exactly why your doctor wants to do it. Informed questioning can help ensure that you undergo only those tests that are absolutely necessary to pinpoint a diagnosis—an accurate one at that. Ask your doctor:

- What are you looking for with this test?
- What are the possible risks of this test?
- What could be the benefits?
- How long does it take to do?
- Does it hurt?
- What will happen to me if I don't have this test or procedure?

Then, based on the answers and ensuing discussion, make the best decision you can.

Q: **I have a sense now of how rheumatoid arthritis affects the joints. But you said earlier that rheumatoid arthritis can affect your whole body. How does it do that?**

A: First, inflammation anywhere in your body can cause an array of body-wide symptoms—fatigue, slight fever, loss of appetite and weight loss. These are some of the earliest symptoms of rheumatoid arthritis, and practically everyone with RA has these symptoms during a flare-up.

Second, rheumatoid arthritis can cause inflammation not only in your joints but anywhere else in your body. Remember, though, that not everyone with RA develops inflammation in other parts of their body. But some do.

Q: **How many?**

A: It's difficult to get a precise number, but according to Arthur Grayzel, M.D., of the Arthritis Foundation, it's "probably less than 10 percent. There is no overall figure quoted in the medical literature on this. Indeed, none of the three major review articles on this topic offer figures. We know only that a certain percentage of people with RA develop certain additional problems, such as rheumatoid nodules."

Q: Will I know if I have inflammation elsewhere in my body?

A: Not always. Many people with this condition never have symptoms, although signs of inflammation are evident at autopsy. "These disorders can develop quickly, but usually they are seen several years into the disease," explains Dr. Hochberg.

Rheumatoid arthritis can inflame blood vessels, a condition called **vasculitis** that can show up as small brown spots or splinter-shaped marks at the base of your fingernails. Vasculitis can cause a number of serious skin problems. People with RA also tend to bruise easily and to develop small **hemorrhages** under their skin—tiny bluish-purple spots.

Some people with RA develop inflammation around their heart, a condition called **pericarditis**, which can range from mild and fleeting to life-threatening. Chest pain, labored breathing and swollen feet and hands are the most common symptoms. A very sensitive test to detect pericarditis is an **echocardiogram**, which uses sound waves to detect fluid around the heart sac and other heart abnormalities.

Other complications of RA include lung problems that make breathing difficult; inflamed nerves (**neuritis**) that can cause loss of sensation in the feet or hands, or muscle paralysis that makes the foot or hand floppy; **carpal tunnel syndrome**, in which nerves in the wrist are compressed; eye problems, including dryness, inflammation and pain; blood and immune-system disorders; and muscle **atrophy**, weakness and tremor.

Q: You mentioned rheumatoid nodules a couple of times. What are these?

A: Rheumatoid nodules, which develop in about 20 percent of people with RA, are tender bumps that tend to form at pressure points around joints—where you might rest your elbows on a table, for instance, or around your tailbone. Generally, nodules don't cause pain. Sometimes, though, they become infected and are treated with antibiotics or drained.

Q: What's the worst rheumatoid arthritis can get?

A: Well, first the bad news. Rheumatoid arthritis isn't the benign condition many doctors once thought it was. That's partly why they are more likely nowadays to treat it aggressively earlier on. Further, no doctor can predict what's going to happen to each individual person. But they know, from population studies, that after 10 to 12 years more than 80 percent of people with rheumatoid arthritis show signs of disability or deformity. They can't move their joints through the full range of motion, their walking is slowed, and perhaps they even have trouble maintaining a grip.

Q: Is there any good news?

A: Yes. Population studies also show that fewer than 5 percent of people with RA become wheelchair-bound or unable to take care of themselves. Most can take care of themselves, even though they have some degree of difficulty, for example, lifting, kneeling, walking, cooking or holding a pen, paintbrush or comb—activities of daily living. Many doctors believe earlier treatment could help prevent permanent joint deformity, since much of this seems to occur within the first few years of the disease.

Q: So it's not going to kill me, right?

A: Very unlikely, but population studies show that, on average, people with rheumatoid arthritis tend to die five to seven years sooner than people without RA, according to Dr. Hochberg. That shortened life span is due to a number of mostly preventable health problems.

Q: What problems?

A: Infections top the list. Even when not taking drugs that suppress the immune system, people with RA have a somewhat weakened immune system caused by the disease itself. So they're more likely to develop serious infections, such as pneumonia, which can kill them, Dr. Hochberg says.

They're also more likely than normal to develop non-Hodgkin's **lymphoma**. This is cancer of the lymph glands, which are part of the immune system.

Dr. Hochberg explains the connection: "Researchers hypothesize that people with RA are at higher risk for these types of cancer because of the immune-system abnormalities associated with RA. Over time, the cells of the immune system lose control over normal proliferation and become malignant."

Q: Now that's really bad news. How frequent is this occurrence?

A: These kinds of cancer are very rare, even in people with RA. Statistics from the National Cancer Institute show that these cancers strike fewer than 1 in 10,000 in the general population, and arthritis researchers think they strike fewer than 3 in 10,000 RA sufferers.

Q: Anything else?

A: Yes. People with RA are more likely to develop stomach and intestinal problems, especially irritation or ulcers caused by anti-inflammatory drugs and other drugs used to treat RA. They may also develop heart or lung problems due to inflammation, and kidney and liver problems, mostly from toxicity to drugs. Dr. Felson, of the Boston University Arthritis Center, and others estimate that "at least 20 to 30 percent of people with RA develop drug-related problems." Unfortunately, there are no good figures on the number of people with RA who develop heart or lung problems from RA-related inflammation, but the incidence of symptom-causing problems is thought to be fairly low—less than 10 percent, according to the Arthritis Foundation.

Q: **But you said there are ways to avoid or prevent the factors associated with a shorter life span. What are some?**

A: Annual flu vaccines, for starters, and a regular vaccine against pneumonia.

Other preventive-health-care activities are also important, because having to take drugs both for arthritis and for another chronic condition, such as high blood pressure or heart disease, is hard on your kidneys. That means being checked regularly for high blood pressure and high cholesterol and having appropriate tests for early cancer detection, such as mammograms and colon examinations. Non-Hodgkin's lymphomas are usually detected as lymph-node or spleen enlargement during a physical examination, or the development of abnormal proteins in the blood.

Preventive care also means taking care of yourself: no smoking or heavy drinking, getting some exercise, maintaining proper weight, eating nutritiously, and perhaps even taking some vitamin supplements. There's research to show that all these self-care tactics can pay off. If you don't smoke or drink, for instance, you're less likely to develop the ulcers or liver damage that sometimes occur as a side effect of certain arthritis drugs. If you exercise, your joints stay healthier and more flexible. And if you maintain your proper weight, you're less likely to have painful osteoarthritis on top of RA.

Q: **Any other preventive "must dos" and no-nos?**

A: Yes, and we'll have more to say about these and other self-care techniques in chapter 5.

Q: But isn't my doctor supposed to closely monitor my disease?

A: Yes, self-care is just one aspect of the equal-partner relationship you should have with a competent practitioner. And indeed, it is crucial to be monitored by a specialist for potentially serious side effects caused by any drugs you may be taking for RA.

The next chapter tells you when it's important to see an arthritis specialist and details the drug and surgical treatments doctors can offer you.

3 ARTHRITIS TREATMENTS (Doctors, Drugs, Surgery)

Q: What kind of treatments are available for people with arthritis?

A: Drugs, physical therapy, occupational therapy, psychological counseling and surgery (not to mention alternative treatments, which we discuss in the next chapter) are all used to treat arthritis.

Q: What treatment offers the best chance to cure arthritis?

A: There's no treatment that cures arthritis, at least not rheumatoid arthritis or osteoarthritis. (Infectious arthritis is another story. It often responds to a single treatment—antibiotics.)

Q: So what does any treatment do, if it doesn't cure?

A: Medical care focuses on relieving pain and reducing inflammation, slowing the progress of the disease, preventing permanent joint damage, improving the function of a joint through surgery if necessary, and keeping the patient and her joints functional throughout her lifetime.

Usually, there's no single treatment that accomplishes all those objectives for any one person. Most people eventually find that a combination of therapies works for them. For some people, aspirin, exercise and vitamin E work, while for others **gold salts**, hot baths and fish oil do the trick. And for still others, none of these remedies work.

DOCTORS

Q: When should you see a doctor about joint or muscle pain?

A: If your aches and pains are not severe and last just a few days, chances are pretty good you don't have arthritis, experts agree. But if your pain persists for more than a few days, recurs over the course of a few weeks or is severe enough to interfere with normal everyday activities, it's time to see a doctor. That's the consensus of opinion, says Herbert Kaplan, M.D., medical director of the Denver Arthritis Clinic and chairman of a committee of doctors that helps develop patient materials for the American College of Rheumatology.

"It's hard to put an exact time frame on it, but if you have an unexplained pain that is compromising your lifestyle or interfering with your sleep, it's time to get some advice from a doctor," he says. Swelling around one or more joints usually means there is an underlying problem. So does symmetrical joint pain or joint pain accompanied by fatigue.

Don't be lulled into complacency if over-the-counter drugs such as aspirin or **ibuprofen** keep your joint pain at bay. If you're using a painkiller regularly and your pain returns when you stop, "it's time to find out what you're treating," Dr. Kaplan says.

Q: What happens if I delay going to a doctor for treatment? Will I become crippled?

A: You could. "If you have an infection in a joint and it goes untreated, you can have permanent, disabling cartilage damage in as little as two weeks," says Joseph Markenson, M.D., an arthritis specialist at the Hospital for Special Surgery in New York City. An infected joint becomes hot and swollen. "If you have such symptoms in a joint or joints, you should see a doctor within hours to a day or so after the condition begins," Dr. Markenson says.

Q: What about rheumatoid arthritis?
Will I become crippled if I delay treatment?

A: Most doctors now think that your chances of
developing permanent joint deformities increase
the longer you delay treatment.

Doctors now know permanent joint damage often occurs
early on—sometimes within weeks to months of the onset of
symptoms. That damage occurs as proliferating synovial tissue
invades the cartilage in the joint, causing the cartilage to
erode. Once that damage has occurred, it cannot be reversed.

That's why many doctors now believe it's important to
begin drug treatment early in the course of the disease. We'll
soon discuss this in more detail.

Q: What about osteoarthritis?
Is early treatment as critical?

A: There's no clear evidence that early treatment helps
osteoarthritis, but you can learn some things to help
you protect and prolong the life of your afflicted joints,
Dr. Kaplan says. "I see a lot of people who think the way to
treat this sort of pain is to 'work it out'—to run up and down
stairs and jog on a painful knee or hip. I am constantly referring people with osteoarthritis to physical therapists, who
teach them better than I could how not to abuse their joints."
Appropriate exercise, joint-protecting **splints** and anti-
inflammatory drugs may help avert the kind of joint injury
that leads to permanent disability.

Q: So seeing a doctor sooner rather than later may
be beneficial. But whom should I see for my
symptoms—my pain and stiffness? How do I
know what kind of doctor is best?

A: Don't panic. First things first. Let's talk about which
doctors can treat joint pain. If you're like most
people, you will first consult your **primary-care physician**
—the doctor you see most of the time for most general ail-
ments. That may be a family doctor or general practitioner.

Both are trained to handle minor illnesses and to recognize a possible serious illness that requires the expertise of a specialist, although a recent study suggests that a primary-care doctor may be slow in recognizing the symptoms of rheumatoid arthritis. (We'll talk more about that study in a bit.)

Sometimes people have an internist as their primary-care doctor. This doctor has an additional three years of medical training in the diagnosis and nonsurgical treatment of diseases, especially those of adults. She can provide long-term comprehensive care in a hospital or her office, managing both common illnesses and complex problems. Some internists specialize in arthritis, as you'll see below.

Whichever doctor you see first should examine your joints carefully and gently, check for other symptoms (such as fever and enlarged lymph glands), ask lots of questions about the onset of your pain and order some of the tests we mentioned earlier.

Q: Will my primary-care physician be the only doctor I see for treatment? Will he ever refer me to a specialist?

A: Your primary-care doctor should refer you to a specialist if he thinks you have a serious illness that he can't diagnose and treat. He may also refer you to a specialist if he is uncertain of your diagnosis. Whether or not your primary-care doctor refers you to a specialist may depend on a number of factors, including your own wishes, the availability of a specialist in your area, even "local politics," Dr. Kaplan admits. "A doctor who feels he's had his patients stolen by a specialist may stop making referrals to that specialist," he says.

Q: How can I determine for myself when I need to see a specialist, even though my primary-care doctor doesn't refer me to one?

A: As with many other areas of medicine calling for consumer savvy, you've got to ask questions, stay informed and evaluate your own symptoms and progress.

"Ask your doctors questions," Dr. Markenson says. "What is my diagnosis? Exactly what type of arthritis do I have? How did you arrive at the diagnosis? What makes you think it's this type and not that?" Your doctor's answers can help you decide whether or not his diagnosis was arrived at in a logical manner.

If your primary-care doctor hasn't given you a clear diagnosis within two to three visits over the course of a few weeks, or if you think his diagnosis is wrong, it's time to see a specialist, Dr. Markenson says. And see a specialist if your primary-care doctor has diagnosed your condition but you don't feel better within four to six months of starting treatment, he adds.

Q: What kind of specialist should I see?

A: A primary-care doctor is most likely to refer a patient with arthritis to either a rheumatologist or an **orthopedist**. A person who appears to have rheumatoid arthritis or some other sort of rheumatic disease is most likely to be referred to a rheumatologist initially. She may be referred to an orthopedist later, if she develops joint problems that would benefit from surgery.

Someone with osteoarthritis may be treated by any one of several kinds of doctors—a primary-care doctor, a rheumatologist, an internist or an orthopedist. She is especially likely to be referred to an orthopedist if she needs joint surgery, although an orthopedist may treat a person with osteoarthritis who doesn't require surgery.

Q: What's a rheumatologist?

A: A rheumatologist is a doctor—either an internist or pediatrician—who specializes in the treatment of diseases of the joints, muscles, bones and tendons. A rheumatologist diagnoses and treats arthritis, back pain, muscle strains, common athletic injuries and diseases of the connective tissues. A rheumatologist may also work closely

with other specialists, such as physical therapists and orthopedic surgeons.

There are about 3,000 rheumatologists in the United States, according to the American College of Rheumatology (ACR). But not all of the 3,000 rheumatologists see patients. Some are involved strictly in research. Like many medical specialists, rheumatologists are in demand, according to Lynn Bonfiglio, membership director for the ACR.

Q: Does that mean I'm going to have to wait weeks to see one?

A: Maybe, depending on where you live, the number of specialists in town or any number of factors.

"My own thinking is that a patient should be seen when she wishes to be seen," Dr. Markenson says. "If a doctor doesn't have an appointment within the next week or two, her own doctor should call and ask him to move the appointment up if he thinks it's important. You shouldn't have to wait a month to see a doctor, especially if your symptoms are getting worse."

Q: What exactly does the specialty training of a rheumatologist involve?

A: Besides four years of medical school and three of residency training in either internal medicine or pediatrics, a rheumatologist has an additional two to three years of specialized training called a fellowship. During that time, she is working in a special arthritis unit or department of a hospital with doctors who have many years of experience treating people with arthritis, explains Ronald Anderson, M.D., director of the rheumatology training program at Brigham and Women's Hospital in Boston.

"It's basically an apprenticeship, with lots of hands-on training," he says. A doctor learns how to diagnose the many kinds of arthritis, becomes familiar with the drugs available for treatment, and may take courses in immunology, molecular biology, bone metabolism and orthopedics, among many other areas.

Q: What's a rheumatologist going to do for me?

A: Because of her training and experience, a rheumatologist knows exactly what questions need to be answered and what tests need to be done in order to make an accurate diagnosis. She is also very familiar with the arsenal of drugs used to treat arthritis, and so can prescribe them appropriately and monitor their side effects.

Since a rheumatologist often works with a team of health-care professionals, she can help to coordinate most aspects of your medical care, including physical therapy.

In a survey of 1,051 arthritis sufferers, done by the authors of the book *Arthritis: What Works* (New York: St. Martin's, 1989), rheumatologists stood out as the reigning experts on the disease and most aspects of its treatment. Half of the survey participants said a rheumatologist helped them find dramatic long-term relief. And 85 percent got at least temporary relief.

Q: How do I find a competent rheumatologist?

A: The most obvious course is to ask your primary-care doctor for a referral. (And ask him *why* he's referring you to a particular doctor. Is it because he's the best rheumatologist in town? The only one? A golfing buddy?)

If you don't have a primary-care doctor, or don't want to ask him, you can call your county medical society for a list of rheumatologists in your area. Or you can call the nearest university hospital. Find out the name of the doctor who heads the rheumatology division. Call him or her and ask for a recommendation.

You can also call your local chapter of the Arthritis Foundation for the names of rheumatologists practicing near you. Get the number from your phone book, county medical society or from the national headquarters of the Arthritis Foundation, 1314 Spring St. N.W., Atlanta, GA 30309; (404) 872-7100.

If you're really stuck, call or write the American College of Rheumatology, 17 Executive Park Dr., Suite 480, Atlanta, GA 30329; (404) 633-3777. Although they normally provide services only to doctors, they can tell you the names of some doctors in your area who are board-certified in rheumatology.

Q: Board-certified? What does that mean?

A: Board certification in rheumatology means that, besides four years of medical school and three years of residency training, a doctor has completed a two-to-three-year fellowship training program in arthritis and has passed a rigorous examination given by the American Board of Internal Medicine (ABIM). A doctor who is board-certified, in effect, has been deemed worthy by his peers of practicing in a particular area of medicine.

Most—but not all—rheumatologists are board-certified in both internal medicine and rheumatology. While board certification is not a guarantee of competent and quality care, it is as good an indication as you're likely to find.

Doctors certified since 1990 need to pass a recertification examination every 10 years in order to remain board-certified.

Q: What about "board eligible"? I've seen that after doctors' names.

A: Some doctors who treat arthritis are board eligible. That means they have completed an accredited fellowship program but have not yet taken—or passed—their board-certification examination. (Exams are given every two years.) "If you don't pass your board after two tries, then in order to qualify to take the boards, you must have had additional education experience in a training program," according to Dr. Anderson. A doctor must also have the recommendation of her teachers before she can take the board-certification examination.

Most rheumatologists who are board-certified also become "fellows" of the American College of Rheumatology, the highest membership category in this specialty's professional organization. To become a fellow, a board-certified doctor must be sponsored by two doctors who are already members of the ACR, and be elected by the ACR's board of directors.

Some older doctors who treat arthritis may have been practicing medicine before board certification in rheumatology was established in 1972. Those doctors were not required to take the boards, although many of them did. Those who did not take the boards are not board certified; nevertheless, many are fellows in the American College of Rheumatology. These older doctors were brought in through recommendations by colleagues who already are fellows in the college.

Q: **Rheumatologists can't all be perfect, though, right?**

A: Well, no. Some of the Arthritis Survey participants—done by the authors of *Arthritis: What Works*—said their rheumatologists did not acknowledge the impact of the side effects of the drugs they were taking. Rashes, diarrhea, nausea and depression were seen as par for the course—something to be expected and lived with—in the mind of the rheumatologists, not a reason to discontinue a drug.

And others said some rheumatologists were rigidly opposed to the possibility of dietary or nutritional help for arthritis because they thought it smacked of quackery. So they're often no help to a patient who wants to explore options outside of mainstream medical practice.

And, like all doctors, there may be rheumatologists who are abrasive, impatient and incompetent. But as we said earlier, for the most part they score high when it comes to providing help.

Q: **Okay, so now I know something about rheumatologists. What can you tell me about orthopedists?**

A: An orthopedist, also called an orthopedic surgeon, is an M.D. or D.O. who specializes in the surgical treatment of bone and joint diseases, deformities and fractures, including all kinds of problems associated with osteo- and rheumatoid arthritis.

He has five years of post-medical-school training in the diagnosis and treatment of diseases and injuries that affect the bones and joints. This doctor is trained to repair bone fractures, cartilage tears, injured muscles, tendons or ligaments, and some joint-associated nerve problems.

Q: Wait a minute—it sounds like all this doctor does is cut and slash. Is that the case?

A: No, orthopedists do more than operate, although when it comes to joint surgery, they're the experts. Some orthopedists do use nonsurgical methods to treat people with arthritis, especially people with osteoarthritis, and can provide a full spectrum of treatment options, including drugs and exercise. In fact, a number of people in the Arthritis Survey said their sole doctor was an orthopedist. They also reported that orthopedists were as likely as rheumatologists to provide dramatic long-term relief.

But a problem often associated with surgical specialists is their tendency to be quick with the scalpel when nonsurgical options are available and possibly more appropriate. For that reason, Dr. Kaplan suggests that anyone whose orthopedist has recommended joint surgery see a rheumatologist for a second opinion.

"A rheumatologist is most familiar with possible nonsurgical options and can suggest those a patient has not tried," he says. "It's not unusual for us to see a patient considering surgery who has not had a proper course of treatment with nonsurgical means, such as anti-inflammatory drugs, joint protection (with splints, for example) or rest."

And even if surgery is the recommended course of treatment, a second surgical opinion is beneficial. Because arthritis is incurable, the range of opinions, even by doctors in the same specialty, often vary widely.

Q: How can I find an orthopedist?

A: If you need to find an orthopedic surgeon, ask your primary-care doctor for a referral. Or call the department of orthopedic surgery at the largest hospital near you or at the closest university-affiliated hospital. Ask the head of the department to recommend a doctor in your area, or if one is not nearby, the next closest locale where a good physician is available. You may also want to call your local office of the Arthritis Foundation (in the white pages of your phone book) or check the yellow pages of your phone book under "Physicians." You can also check the doctor-referral services operated by your county medical society.

If you and your doctors determine that surgery is necessary, your best bet is to have the surgery done by an orthopedic surgeon affiliated with a hospital rheumatology department, who's likely to operate on many people with arthritis. You may be able to find that doctor at a large university hospital in your region. Or check in the list in the back of this book to see if you live near one of the 14 multipurpose arthritis centers associated with the National Institute of Arthritis and Musculoskeletal and Skin Diseases.

Make sure you choose a doctor who performs the operation you're to have many times a year, whether it's a total joint replacement or shaving off a bit of rough cartilage. "If your surgeon replaces only a few joints a year, you may have a higher likelihood of infection or poor fit of an artificial joint," Dr. Markenson says.

If you live in a small town, it may be impossible to find an orthopedic surgeon who does the kind of surgery you require often enough to have the kind of expertise you might like, Dr. Markenson admits. "Some of this surgery is technically difficult, even for surgeons who do it all the time," he says. "You want someone who's comfortable doing it."

Some doctors recommend that at least 60 percent of a surgeon's practice consist of joint-replacement operations. Some experts even suggest 75 percent as a minimum. "I can't tell you exactly how many joint-replacement operations a surgeon should do in a year to remain proficient, but I think you should ask the surgeon you are considering how many he does," says Dr. Markenson. At the Hospital for Special Surgery in New York City, a surgeon specializing in this operation does an average of 150 joint replacements a year.

"And it's not unreasonable to look for a medical center that replaces 1,200 joints a year," advises Dr. Markenson. At the Hospital for Special Surgery in New York City, for example, 2,200 joint replacements are performed yearly.

Q: What other doctors treat arthritis?

A: Just about any kind of doctor may treat one or another symptom of arthritis, so we'll stick with those doctors most commonly used.

Osteopaths, also called Doctors of Osteopathy, or D.O.'s, are fully licensed physicians and surgeons whose medical training is basically the same as an M.D.'s. As a general rule, though, D.O.'s tend to be more holistic than M.D.'s in their approach to care. "They focus on the patient, not the disease, and hold that the body is an interrelated system," explains David Bevan, D.O., chairman of the division of rheumatology at the Philadelphia College of Osteopathic Medicine.

The practitioners are called *osteo*paths because they emphasize the role of bones, muscles and joints of the body—the musculoskeletal system—in a person's well-being. Consequently, manipulation and hands-on diagnosis and treatment are the mainstays of osteopathic practice, Dr. Bevan explains.

An osteopathic doctor can use palpation (touch), literally a hands-on diagnostic procedure, to detect soft-tissue changes or structural abnormalities. D.O.'s also use manipulative therapy, whereby muscles, bones, joints, nerves and tissue have pressure applied to them in order to effect some beneficial change in a patient's condition.

But osteopaths also use the same drugs and surgery that M.D.'s use, if and when such treatment is necessary.

Some osteopaths have specialized training in rheumatology, sometimes in the same programs as medical doctors. They can be board-certified in internal medicine through the American Osteopathic Association. Most are general practitioners, however.

In the Arthritis Survey, participants said osteopaths were about as effective as allopathic general practitioners or family doctors at relieving their arthritis pain. The doctors provided at least moderate relief to slightly more than half of the people they saw. People also say these doctors were very helpful at providing advice and guidance on exercise and other nondrug, nonsurgical alternatives, such as heat, cold and nutrition.

A physiatrist (*not* psychiatrist) is an M.D. who specializes in physical medicine and rehabilitation, the medical specialty concerned with diagnosing, evaluating and treating patients with impairments or disabilities that involve the muscles and skeleton, nerves and other body systems.

Such doctors are trained to devise preventive or rehabilitative exercise programs, and are also likely to be familiar with nondrug and nonsurgical treatments for arthritis. Those treatments include splinting, exercise, water therapy (such as whirlpools), ice, heat, movement, ultrasound and electrical stimulation, explains Valery Lanyi, M.D., a physiatrist and associate clinical professor of medicine at New York University Medical Center.

Physiatrists may also use a treatment called *trigger-point therapy*. In this form of treatment a local painkiller or a saline solution is injected into a painful area of a damaged muscle. The injections sometimes stop the pain. ''These injections are not used for arthritis per se, but they may be used for muscle problems in the neck or lower back that are associated with arthritis,'' Dr. Lanyi says.

Q: When should I see a physiatrist rather than another practitioner?

A: The answer depends a lot upon whom you talk to. Obviously, physiatrists believe they have much to offer people with arthritis.

Generally speaking, someone whose ability to function has been impaired may benefit from a consultation with a physiatrist. So might people considering surgery on a joint, who have multiple joint involvement, or who are having problems using their hands. A physiatrist can devise a specialized exercise program, use nondrug treatments to relieve pain, and make up immobilizing splints for inflamed joints to help prevent permanent damage.

Many physiatrists work with physical and **occupational therapists**, some of whom specialize in certain parts of the body, such as the hands or feet.

Q: Are there any other specialists I should know about?

A: A neurologist, a doctor who diagnoses and treats disorders of the nerves, may be called in—by a specialist, such as a rheumatologist, or even a primary-care physician—to assess nerve damage caused by arthritis. And a neurosurgeon may be called in to perform surgery on your neck or back. She might remove osteoarthritic bone spurs on your spine that are pinching nerves in your back, for instance, or fuse together damaged vertebrae to give your spine added stability.

Q: Whew—that's quite a variety of options. Family doctors, rheumatologists, orthopedists, even physiatrists and neurologists treat arthritis. Any other practitioners?

A: Yes, chiropractors and allergists may also get into the act, but they are considered alternatives, or adjuncts, to the practitioners we've discussed in this section. We'll explore the options in alternative care in the next chapter.

Q: Do people spend a lot of time looking for help?

A: You bet they do. In the Arthritis Survey, most of the 1,051 participants consulted at least 2 or 3 medical specialists for help, and some of them saw as many as 9 or 10. The searching apparently paid off, because about two-thirds said they were satisfied with their current care. Along the way, however, both patient and doctor are likely to make some mistakes.

Q: Mistakes? Like what?

A:
Doctors, especially nonspecialists, can take a long time to come up with a diagnosis, says Dr. Felson, of the Boston University Arthritis Center.

While it's true that arthritis can be difficult to diagnose in its early stages, Dr. Felson and fellow researchers who studied the subject found that primary-care doctors still took more than six months to diagnose one out of five patients with classic, obvious signs of rheumatoid arthritis—symmetrical joint pain, morning stiffness and a positive blood test for rheumatoid factor.

"The point we're trying to make is that primary-care doctors may not be as aware as they ought to be when it comes to recognizing the symptoms of rheumatoid arthritis, and they might not refer to a specialist as rapidly as they need to," Dr. Felson says. "In fact, it's frequently *not* your primary-care doctor who makes the diagnosis—he winds up eventually referring you to a specialist. Or if he does figure out the diagnosis, it takes 3½ months until that happens. We think that's too long."

Q: So what can someone do about that?

A:
"Make your primary-care doctor aware that you are concerned that you may have some kind of arthritis, and have him investigate it," Dr. Felson recommends.

Q: Do doctors make any other mistakes?

A:
Once they've finally diagnosed arthritis, the next mistake some doctors make is to undertreat it—not take it seriously enough to provide effective treatment or suggest a doctor who can. To minimize the harm done you as a result of such a mistake, it's important to have medical care from a specialist.

Q: Do people with arthritis make mistakes?

A: Some patients themselves make the mistake of waiting *years* to see a mainstream doctor about their symptoms, Dr. Markenson says.

Q: Why would they do that?

A: No one knows for sure. It may be that their symptoms were very mild, or that they thought their symptoms were an inevitable consequence of growing older and nothing to see a doctor about. Or it may also be that they sought help outside of mainstream medicine first—at least according to many doctors, traditional practitioners themselves, who may be biased against anything outside the mainstream.

"A study done a few years ago asked just that question—why people took so long to seek treatment for arthritis," Dr. Markenson says. "The people answering the question had a number of choices. It turns out that those who stay away from doctors the longest—an average of four years from the onset of their symptoms—are those who are using a quack cure. We don't know if it was helping them, or if they thought there was nothing else they could do, but it was sure keeping them out of a doctor's office."

Q: Okay, let's recap this. The best way for me to get appropriate medical care is . . . ?

A:
• If you have joint pain or swelling that persists, see a doctor.

• Start with your family doctor, general practitioner or internist.

• If your family doctor, general practitioner or internist is not able to diagnose your condition in two or three visits over the course of a few weeks, see a specialist.

• Also see a specialist if the treatment your primary-care doctor offers has not provided relief within four to six months, or see one immediately if your symptoms get worse.

DRUGS

Q: You've indicated that a number of practitioners, notably family doctors, rheumatologists and internists, use drugs to treat arthritis. Is this the primary treatment mode?

A: Yes. In conjunction with exercise and rest, heat, cold and other physical therapies, drugs are a mainstay of treatment for both rheumatoid arthritis and osteoarthritis. Drugs help relieve pain and inflammation, and, in the case of rheumatoid arthritis, may help prevent joint damage.

Q: What kinds of drugs are used to treat arthritis?

A: There are several different types. Doctors usually divide them into *first-line* and *second-line* drugs.
The first-line drugs are usually—not always—tried first and include **nonsteroidal anti-inflammatory drugs (NSAIDs)**, such as aspirin, ibuprofen and an array of prescription drugs. These drugs are used for both osteoarthritis and rheumatoid arthritis. First-line drugs used almost exclusively for the treatment of rheumatoid arthritis also include **steroid drugs**, such as prednisone and **cortisone**, although, because of side effects, these drugs really *aren't* a first choice. Steroid drugs are seldom used for osteoarthritis because they are not helpful for this condition and have potentially serious side effects.
Because they are not effective in the treatment of osteoarthritis, second-line drugs are used to treat only rheumatoid arthritis. They are also sometimes called **disease-modifying** or disease-remittive drugs because their use seems to bring on a remission of symptoms in many people. These drugs include gold salts, as shots or pills; **Plaquenil**, or **hydroxychloroquine**, a drug also used to treat malaria; **penicillamine**, a cousin of the famous antibiotic; and **methotrexate** and other **immunosuppressive** drugs also used to treat cancer.

Q: Hmmm. Sounds mind boggling. How do doctors figure out what drugs to use?

A: This is something doctors spend a long time learning, partly by clinical research and partly by instinct. As one doctor puts it, "There's no cookbook." Which drugs work best for which people is pretty much of an art, admits James E. Brick, M.D., associate professor of medicine at the West Virginia University School of Medicine. "The role of the rheumatologist is to figure out which drugs will do a patient the most good with the least harm," he says.

A lot of variables go into that equation, Dr. Brick emphasizes. "How old the patient is, how active, what other kinds of medical problems he has, whether he is willing to take some risks with a newer drug or wants to stick with an older, better-studied drug, how he has reacted to drugs given earlier, how his disease seems to be progressing, what kinds of monitoring tests he is willing to put up with: Those kinds of things all need to be considered before you decide how to treat someone."

Some people who have a particularly aggressive form of RA by the time they get to the doctor, for instance, may be put directly on a second-line drug. "A doctor's choice of drugs is based upon both the severity of the disease and the stage of the disease at presentation," says Jon D. Levine, M.D., Ph.D., professor of medicine at the University of California School of Medicine in San Francisco. "If you show up in my office for the first time with many inflamed joints, and x-rays show you already have signs of joint destruction, I would probably prescribe a second-line drug immediately, and perhaps also give an NSAID for its analgesic effect."

Another thing doctors and patients alike need to keep in mind is that a majority of people with arthritis do okay on just about any arthritis drug, initially. But after a few years, it's not uncommon for the drug to stop working so well, or for it to begin to cause troubling side effects. In either case, it's on to another drug or a combination of drugs. "In patients who are being treated for a long time, at some point it becomes a juggling act," Dr. Brick explains. "You try to make them feel as good as you can, as long as you can, without killing them with the medicine."

Q: Oh, great. Well, I guess I better learn something about these drugs. Let's start with the first-line drugs. What are nonsteroidal anti-inflammatory drugs?

A: As the name indicates, NSAIDs (pronounced EN-seds) are drugs that fight inflammation—pain, swelling, heat and redness. They do that by blocking biochemicals in the body, called **prostaglandins**, some of which cause inflammation. By the way, NSAIDs are distinguished from steroid drugs, which also relieve pain and inflammation, by the fact that they work in an entirely different manner and have very different side effects.

NSAIDs include a few different groups of drugs: aspirin (acetylsalicylate) and related compounds (salicylamide, salsalate), ibuprofen (as found in Advil or Nuprin) and more than a dozen other chemical compounds. If your doctor suggests one NSAID and it doesn't work, he's likely then to have you try one in a different chemical group.

Q: Do you mean that simple aspirin can actually help my arthritis?

A: It very well might. For many kinds of arthritis, including rheumatoid arthritis and osteoarthritis, NSAIDs are a first-line treatment, and from among these drugs, aspirin is often selected. According to the Arthritis Survey, many people with arthritis take aspirin, and they say it relieves their painful, swollen joints. And it's inexpensive, compared with other arthritis drugs.

Q: How much aspirin do I need to take?

A: Even though aspirin is available without a prescription, it's important to work with your doctor to figure out just how much you need to take to control your symptoms. You can take too much and will suffer the consequences —ringing ears, fluid retention, even internal bleeding. People with osteoarthritis may need only small amounts of aspirin to control their pain, or they may not even need an NSAID at all.

People with rheumatoid arthritis, on the other hand, often need large amounts to control symptoms of joint inflammation. A doctor may recommend taking three or four standard aspirin tablets four times daily—with meals and a bedtime snack. (A standard tablet contains five grains of aspirin, which is equal to 325 milligrams of the drug. An "extra-strength" or "arthritis-strength" tablet usually contains 500 mg.)

Your doctor should help you figure out the best dosage for you.

Q: What kind of aspirin is best to take?

A: No one kind is best. Aspirin comes in several forms —buffered and enteric-coated—that have been developed to make them more convenient to take and to try to avoid some of the major side effects associated with its use—stomach distress and ulcers. These side effects are more likely to appear with the large dosages recommended for people with rheumatoid arthritis.

Buffered aspirin contains antacidlike ingredients that are supposed to minimize aspirin's stomach-irritating effects. Aspirin with a special coating (called enteric-coated) dissolves only when it reaches your small intestine, so the coating saves your stomach from direct contact with the aspirin. But neither of these forms of aspirin offers complete protection from potentially dangerous side effects, which we'll discuss in a minute.

Both of these forms of aspirin are available in nonbrand-name, or generic, versions, which work just as well as the popular brands and cost a lot less. Buying a bottle of 1,000 generic enteric-coated aspirin tablets may be the least expensive, least stomach-irritating way to go. A quick tip: To keep the tablets fresh, store the bottle in a dry, cool place—not your bathroom!

Q: You said that people with osteoarthritis may not need to take an NSAID. So what kind of drug would they take?

A: Since mild osteoarthritis may involve pain but not inflammation, an anti-inflammatory drug, with all its possible side effects, may not be necessary. People with osteoarthritis may do just fine taking an aspirin substitute, **acetaminophen**, which is found in Tylenol, Datril, Anacin-3 and various other brands.

In fact, when researchers at Indiana University compared how well people with chronic knee pain caused by osteo-arthritis responded to four weeks of treatment with either acetaminophen or the NSAID ibuprofen, they found that a high dose of acetaminophen worked just as well as either a high or low dose of ibuprofen.

These researchers say that with a four- to six-week trial of about 2,000 mg. of acetaminophen a day—about six 325 mg. tablets, and within the normal dosage range—you should know whether this drug relieves your pain. Acetaminophen has few side effects, but in very large doses it can cause serious liver damage.

Q: Aside from aspirin, what other kinds of NSAIDs are available?

A: Many different over-the-counter drugs contain aspirin or related compounds. Some contain ibuprofen, (a.k.a. Motrin or Advil), also a very popular—and effective—arthritis drug.

Many NSAIDs are available by prescription only. Some of those commonly used for arthritis include Motrin (ibuprofen) in dosages up to four times the over-the-counter version, Indocin (indomethacin), Naprosyn (naproxen), Feldene (piroxicam), Tolectin (tolmetin) and Clinoril (sulindac).

Q: Why are these drugs available only by prescription while some other NSAIDs are not?

A: These drugs have potentially serious side effects that require a doctor's monitoring.

Q: Why are so many drugs designed to do basically the same thing—relieve pain and inflammation?

A: Good question. One reason is because drug manufacturers are always trying to come up with new drugs that work as well as, or better than, aspirin but have fewer of the nasty side effects we already mentioned—stomach distress and ulcers. Another reason is that a large selection provides a benefit: Some people fail to respond to a particular NSAID, but when they try a different one, it works.

Q: But are NSAIDs so very different from one another?

A: To hear the pharmaceutical companies' talk, you would think so. Every time a new NSAID hits the market, the drug manufacturer touts this drug as effective (at least as effective as those already on the market) with fewer side effects. The truth so far is that NSAIDs on the market perform pretty much the same, says Dr. Sack, of the University of California at San Francisco.

"Some doctors feel that Motrin is consistently a good actor, that it has the least effects, and they consistently put some other drugs down on the bottom of the list. But there are studies being done on this all the time, and the results are mixed," Dr. Sack says. "You can't say just one drug is great and the others stink."

Q: How soon can I tell if an NSAID is working for me?

A: Your pain and inflammation may not be relieved immediately—it may take a while. Generally, you'll spend a week or two gradually increasing your dosage to get up to a "therapeutic level"—a dosage that maintains the drug at a blood level that should reduce pain and relieve inflammation. Your doctor may want you to continue that dosage for about a month before she and you decide whether the drug is working for you, according to Dr. Brick and others. If it's not working, she'll most likely move on to another NSAID, at least for a while.

Unlike in years past, patients are switched quickly from one NSAID to another if a drug does not seem to be working. And doctors are quicker to move on to second-line drugs if NSAIDs don't bring inflammation under control.

"Nearly every doctor still gives most RA patients a good trial with NSAIDs," Dr. Brick says. "In years past, though, doctors would give NSAIDs for 12 months or longer, or they would wait until a patient had signs of joint erosions on his x-rays, before switching to stronger drugs. You don't see that very much any more. Doctors still use mostly the same drugs, in pretty much the same order as they used to, but the treatment time is contracted now. Most doctors don't wait until they see joint erosions to start people on gold shots. They don't keep patients on NSAIDs who have active inflammation and who are miserable. They go right on to trying something else."

Q: Wait a minute. Before we go on to that something else, I want to know more about the side effects NSAIDs have. What are they?

A: All arthritis drugs have side effects, and the NSAIDs are no exception. Some of these we've already mentioned: stomach irritation (often associated with just about any NSAID, including aspirin), heartburn, indigestion, pain, nausea and vomiting.

And about one in five people who take these drugs in large doses or over a long period of time develops stomach or intestinal ulcers, studies show. That's about 10 times the normal rate.

Q: Ulcers—aren't they sometimes serious?

A: These ulcers are nothing to write off. They may result in 10,000 to 20,000 deaths annually, according to statistics from the U.S. Department of Health and Human Services.

Q: You mean that the aspirin or whatever NSAID I take can dissolve a hole in my stomach?

A: No, these ulcers don't occur only from direct contact of the drug with your stomach or intestines. The ulcers occur because NSAIDs suppress biochemicals in your body called prostaglandins. As you'll recall, we said earlier that some prostaglandins can cause inflammation. But other prostaglandins are good; they help maintain the cells that form your stomach lining. Unfortunately, the NSAIDs suppress both types of prostaglandins.

Q: Sounds serious. What can I do to avoid getting ulcers?

A: Three things if you are taking NSAIDs. Be closely monitored by your doctor for early signs of ulcers; reduce related risk factors, and take a drug that helps to protect against the development of ulcers.

Q: First things first—what kind of monitoring should my doctor do?

A: Every couple of months, your doctor should do a blood test called a CBC (complete blood count). This test can detect a decrease in red blood cells that may mean you are bleeding internally. Your doctor may also have you test your stool for blood. That's a simple at-home test you can do every couple of weeks.

Your doctor should also ask you about stomach pains or any other kind of stomach discomfort—if he doesn't, make sure you volunteer the information. Be aware, though, that pain is not always present with NSAID-induced ulcers, since the drugs themselves can mask the ulcer pain.

You can do something in the way of self-care. Contact your doctor immediately if you vomit blood or develop black, tarry stools. They are signs of internal bleeding. And check with your doctor if you have severe heartburn, stomach pain that goes away after you eat food or take antacids, severe stomach cramps, or occasional nausea or vomiting without any reason.

Q: **How else can I reduce my risk of developing ulcers?**

A: Don't smoke cigarettes, don't drink alcohol and don't take steroid drugs along with NSAIDs. All three up your odds.

Q: **Isn't there a drug to prevent these ulcers?**

A: Yes, it's called Cytotec (misoprostol). This unique drug stimulates the growth of mucus-producing cells that form the stomach. It is currently the only drug approved by the U.S. Food and Drug Administration for use in preventing stomach ulcers in people taking NSAIDs. In clinical trials, people taking NSAIDS who also took either 400 or 800 micrograms of Cytotec daily had a significant reduction in stomach-lining injury compared with a group taking a **placebo** (a harmless blank pill). The rate of microscopic stomach injury was 70 to 75 percent in the placebo group but only 10 to 30 percent in those taking Cytotec.

The most common side effects of Cytotec, diarrhea and abdominal pain, occurred in about 13 percent of people.

This side effect can be minimized by taking the drug right after meals or at bedtime.

This drug is expensive, however. In one East Coast town, the cost of a month's supply of 200 mcg. tablets ranged from about $75 to $100.

"There doesn't seem to be a real consensus among doctors on who needs this drug," says Dr. Grayzel, the Arthritis Foundation's senior vice president for medical affairs. "Most rheumatologists will prescribe it to someone who's had a bleeding ulcer in the past, and some will prescribe it to patients age 60 or older or people with diseases that would make developing an ulcer very risky."

Dr. Grayzel suggests that if you're concerned about ulcers, ask your doctor if he recommends Cytotec.

Q: **What about other, less expensive ulcer drugs? Can't I take them?**

A: Some doctors prescribe other ulcer drugs, such as Tagamet or Zantac (histamine blockers), or strong antacids to their patients taking NSAIDS. These drugs can help heal an ulcer that's already formed if NSAIDs are stopped during the two- to three-month healing process, but there is no proof that they help to stop stomach ulcers from forming, Dr. Grayzel says. "It's not clear how effective these drugs really are, but some doctors prescribe them for symptoms like heartburn."

Q: **Okay—the stomach and intestines can take a beating. What other side effects do NSAIDs have?**

A: A few people develop asthma, hay fever, nasal congestion or hives from aspirin or other NSAIDs. If they develop such symptoms, they should avoid taking drugs containing aspirin or related compounds in the future.

Aspirin and some other NSAIDs can slow blood-clotting time, making bleeding a problem. For this reason, these drugs usually are stopped for one to two weeks prior to any kind of surgery.

High doses of aspirin can make your ears ring and cause slight deafness. Usually this indicates that you've taken too much aspirin for your system; you should reduce your dosage and call your doctor.

Aspirin and other NSAIDs—and many other drugs—can cause fluid retention and problems for your kidneys and liver. If you begin to retain fluid and swell up, gain a lot of weight or feel ill while you're taking one of these drugs, stop taking it and call your doctor pronto! It may mean a drug is building up to a toxic level in your body.

Q: Is toxicity a common problem with these drugs?

A: It can be a problem for some, especially older people and those taking additional drugs, such as diuretics (drugs that flush fluid out of your body). And certain drugs can build up to toxic levels in your body much faster than others, causing kidney or liver damage.

The percentage of people who develop kidney or liver toxicity varies from drug to drug. To check the percentage of people who develop toxicities for the drug you are taking, consult the *Physician's Desk Reference* (Montvale, N.J.: Medical Economics Company), which is published annually and available in many libraries.

Q: Why is toxicity a problem?

A: "Part of the reason is that many of the newer, potent anti-inflammatory drugs, such as Feldene, are available only in a fixed dosage," explains Charles F. Seifert, Pharm. D., associate professor at the University of Oklahoma College of Pharmacy. "Because of that, doctors don't measure blood levels of the drug. Nor do they determine the correct dosage based on a person's weight and age."

Result? A 100-pound woman takes the same amount of the drug as a 240-pound fullback. It's the small woman who's likely to suffer the side effects.

Q: What can I do about this problem?

A: Get regular urine and blood tests that can detect kidney and liver damage. If the tests indicate you are developing problems, your doctor should change you to a different drug in the same class, at a lower equivalent dosage.

Q: Are NSAIDs the only first-line drugs?

A: No. Steroid drugs are called first-line drugs, too, but that's something of a misnomer. These drugs are not likely to be the first choice for most kinds of arthritis, and they are almost never used for osteoarthritis.

Q: Why? Are steroids really dangerous to take?

A: They can be. Steroids were once given in large doses, for long periods of time, for inflammation-producing diseases like rheumatoid arthritis. Because they were used in large doses for long amounts of time, they produced many side effects: lowered resistance to infection, weight gain, "moon face," bone loss, muscle wasting, mood changes, blurred vision, cataracts, diabetes and increased blood pressure, to name a few.

These days, for most cases of rheumatoid arthritis, steroids are generally not used in large amounts, or for very long, so serious side effects are less likely to occur, Dr. Grayzel says. Still, these drugs do need to be used carefully, to make sure they are not causing the above-mentioned side effects.

Q: What exactly are steroids?

A: Steroids are synthetic copies of inflammation-taming hormones, called corticosteroids and glucocorticoids, produced by the body's adrenal glands. The drugs go by such names as dexamethasone, hydrocortisone and prednisone.

Q: How are steroids prescribed?

A: Doctors seem to vary widely in how they prescribe steroids.

"You are going to find some doctors who think steroids are just terrible for patients and others who think they should be used for everything," Dr. Sack says. "Doctors use different dosages and keep patients on them for different amounts of time."

Because oral steroids, such as prednisone, provide almost immediate relief of pain and inflammation, they may be given in addition to NSAIDs to relieve severe symptoms, especially when both patient and doctor are waiting for a slower-acting drug, such as gold, to kick in.

Some doctors also offer their patients steroids to help them get through a flare-up, especially if the patient is the sole breadwinner of a family, so that the person can continue to work.

And some doctors keep patients on low doses of steroids (less than 10 mg. a day) for months or years. "This may include people who aren't responding to NSAIDs and, especially, people who are at high risk of developing side effects from NSAIDs, such as someone who's very old," Dr. Grayzel says. "In someone who's quite old, you would not be so concerned about the long-term consequences of steroid use, such as osteoporosis, which take 10 years or so to develop."

Q: How can I avoid trouble with steroids?

A: Most doctors agree that you should take them in the smallest dose that relieves your symptoms for as short a time as possible.

Further, these drugs need to be tapered off—slowly reduced in dosage—before they are finally stopped altogether. That's because they suppress your body's production of steroids. By reducing the dose slowly, your body has time to come back to normal steroid production.

Most doctors have their patients begin to slowly taper off the drug after eight to twelve weeks of use, or sooner if possible.

Here again, it's important to ask your doctor lots of questions. Why are you prescribing this drug? What are its benefits to me? What are the risks? How can I minimize the risks? How do you intend to monitor for risks?

Q: How does a doctor monitor for steroid risks?

A: Regular blood-pressure checks, a CBC and blood tests that check blood sugar are important. Some doctors also occasionally do an x-ray test that checks bone density.

Q: Are steroids only taken orally?

A: No. Steroids can be injected directly into just about any inflamed joint, and usually provide quick relief that may last for months, even years.

Q: **Is there an advantage to injections rather than oral steroids?**

A: Injections do not cause the body-wide side effects, such as bone loss or lowered resistance to infection, that are seen with oral steroids.

But many doctors caution that a joint should not be injected more than three times a year. Others recommend no more than once every three months. That's because frequently repeated injections are thought to lead to joint destruction.

Another word of caution from experts: Steroids should never be injected into a joint that's infected, because they can make the infection worse. Your doctor should rule out infection by checking the fluid in the joint for signs of infection before she gives you the shot.

Q: **Are steroids ever used to treat osteoarthritis?**

A: Systemic, or oral steroids, have no place in the treatment of osteoarthritis, most experts agree. That's because osteoarthritis seldom involves severe inflammation, the condition steroid drugs treat best. Nevertheless, some doctors believe steroid injections into a painful joint may be given three times a year in severe cases of osteoarthritis, when joints will eventually have to be replaced.

Q: **When do the second-line, or disease-remittive, drugs come in?**

A: As the name implies, a second-line drug—gold, methotrexate and the like—may be added to your treatment if NSAIDs aren't working well enough to relieve your symptoms. As we already stressed, these drugs are reserved almost exclusively for rheumatoid arthritis and other rheumatic diseases and are seldom used for osteoarthritis.

Q: How do second-line drugs differ from first-line drugs?

A: All second-line drugs are slow acting. They can take weeks or months to take effect.

Unlike NSAIDs and steroids, these drugs are thought to slow the progress of your disease. They do sometimes bring on remission or partial remission. In truth, though, there's little scientific evidence to prove that these drugs actually do slow the progress of rheumatoid arthritis. The little proof there is seems to indicate that these drugs have a major impact in slowing the course of rheumatoid arthritis only when they are used early in the development of the disease.

The only clinical trial that supports the theory that second-line drugs can help prevent permanent joint damage was done by Dutch researchers. That study, published in 1989 in the journal *Lancet*, found that a drug used most often for the treatment of ulcerative colitis, **sulfasalazine**, helped to prevent joint-cartilage breakdown in people with early rheumatoid arthritis.

As for anecdotal evidence, doctors point out that people who have aggressive RA often do better than those with slow-acting RA because they are treated sooner with second-line drugs.

Because of these findings, many doctors who treat rheumatoid arthritis now turn to these drugs earlier than they used to. "How soon a doctor turns to a second-line drug depends on several things, including what stage of the disease a patient is in when he first sees the doctor," says Dr. Levine. "Some people may be started on them immediately." Others may be started on second-line drugs if NSAIDS have not controlled their inflammation within three to six months, or if the risk of NSAID-related side effects, such as ulcers, is high, Dr. Levine adds.

Q: But why even bother to be treated with these drugs if there is so little proof that they do anything to slow the course of the disease?

A: "Now you are talking about the major debate of rheumatology," Dr. Levine says. "Are these second-line drugs disease-remitting agents or not? No one knows for sure.'' But while there's a lot of debate about whether or not these drugs have a marked effect of the course of the disease, there's little doubt that many of these drugs provide marked improvement in the quality of life for many people with RA, by relieving symptoms, he adds.

Q: **Tell me again—what are the most commonly prescribed second-line drugs?**

A: These drugs include gold salts, as shots or pills; Plaquenil, or hydroxychloroquine, a drug also used to treat malaria; penicillamine, a cousin of the famous antibiotic; and methotrexate and other immunosuppressive drugs also used to treat cancer.

Q: **You said gold—do you mean the same metal that's used in jewelry? How does it work in the treatment of arthritis?**

A: A form of the same precious metal used in jewelry, gold salts can be given as injections or pills. Gold has been used since the 1920s to treat rheumatoid arthritis, and it works well enough that potential new drugs are always compared with gold to see if they do as well.

Researchers don't know how gold works—it doesn't seem to have much measurable impact on the body's immune system—but it does work. Several researchers have shown that gold relieves pain and inflammation and seems to prevent further deformity in as many as 6 out of 10 people who try it early in the course of their disease. Late starters may also benefit.

Q: **How is gold given?**

A: Gold injections are usually given once a week during the first few months, in slowly increasing doses, then once a month as a maintenance dose.

Oral gold is convenient—no shots! It's usually given as two capsules daily.

Q: What kinds of side effects does gold have?

A: Kidney damage is a possible serious side effect. To detect early signs of kidney injury, urine tests are done repeatedly during therapy.

Damage to the bone marrow (where the body manufactures red and white blood cells and platelets) is another possible serious side effect. To identify this complication, blood tests are done from time to time.

An itchy skin rash can occur, too. Generally, the rash is mild and affects only a few spots on the body. Sometimes, though, it can be severe. The rash usually disappears within a few weeks if gold is stopped.

In about 3 out of 10 people, injectable gold has to be stopped because of some side effect. People taking oral gold are less likely to have the serious side effects that would necessitate stopping the drug, but they still need to be monitored for side effects. And they're more likely to develop diarrhea with oral gold than with gold injections. "Oral gold is thought to be a little safer than gold injections, but it's a little less effective," Dr. Sack says. Some doctors say they are less likely these days than in the past to prescribe oral gold, although injections are still a much-used treatment.

If either form of gold is going to work, you'll feel a clear difference within three to six months, doctors say. One or two people out of every 10 get no benefit from injected gold.

Q: Is gold an expensive treatment?

A: Treatment with gold injections costs an average of $47 a week. That includes the cost of giving the injection. Oral gold costs an average of $12.66 a week, according to figures compiled by Mark Prashkar, M.D., associate professor of medicine at the Boston University Arthritis Center.

Q: You mentioned another second-line drug with a name that sounds a lot like penicillin. What is it? How does it work? How is it different from gold?

A: This drug, called penicillamine, is known to remove copper from the body. That makes it an ideal treatment for people with a rare illness called Wilson's disease, which causes a potentially fatal buildup of copper in the body. But no one knows what penicillamine does to make it effective against the pain and inflammation of rheumatoid arthritis, or if its ability to remove copper is important in this regard. The drug seems to influence the immune system.

In studies, penicillamine seems to work about as well as gold, in the people who can tolerate it. The drug's notorious side effects—kidney problems, rashes, muscle weakness and bone-marrow suppression, along with others—have made it fall out of favor with rheumatologists. "Rheumatologists used to use it a lot in people who had failed to respond to gold injections or couldn't tolerate gold," Dr. Brick says. "Now, though, the place penicillamine occupied in the list of antirheumatic drugs has been largely taken over by the immunosuppressive drugs, such as methotrexate."

Q: Wait a minute. What about the malaria drug you said is also used to treat arthritis. What is it, and how does it work?

A: This drug is called Plaquenil, and, like gold, no one really understands how it works. Also like gold, it takes three to six months to relieve your pain and inflammation. "Plaquenil is not considered as effective as gold, but some doctors like to try this drug before they try gold, because, if it works, their patient is way ahead of the game," Dr. Sack says. "They are likely to be able to stay on it for a long time with few serious side effects." That's because Plaquenil is one of the safest second-line arthritis drugs.

Q: What kind of side effects does Plaquenil have?

A: It has very few side effects on the blood. Its chief worrisome side effect is on the eye, but doctors are now using lower doses that are much less likely to have this effect.

Q: What happens to the eye?

A: Plaquenil can damage the retina, the cells lining the back of the eye, so if you're taking this drug, you need to have your eyes checked every four to six months.

Q: Sorry to keep asking about money, but I've heard that arthritis can be expensive to treat. Is Plaquenil expensive?

A: Treatment with Plaquenil costs about half as much as gold injections. Six months' worth of Plaquenil costs $600, compared to about $1,200 for gold injections.

Q: Now, about these immunosuppressive drugs you've been talking about—what do they do?

A: These drugs make your immune system a little less lively, so, in the case of rheumatoid arthritis, the renegade immune cells that are nibbling at your joints back off a bit. Unfortunately, these drugs affect your *entire* immune system, increasing your risks of developing some serious infections. Plus, they have other potentially life-threatening side effects.

The most popular of these drugs, methotrexate (Rheumatrex) was first used experimentally to treat rheumatoid arthritis in 1951. But it wasn't until recently, after many years of study, that methotrexate was given FDA approval for this use and rheumatologists started using it with some frequency.

These drugs were first used, in doses hundreds of times larger, to treat cancer. They are also used to prevent the rejection of transplanted organs.

Q: When is methotrexate used for rheumatoid arthritis instead of gold or Plaquenil, the antimalarial drug?

A: Some doctors try methotrexate on their patients who have not improved on gold or Plaquenil. Others may suggest either methotrexate or gold injections to a patient and let the patient decide. "These drugs were once used in a more rigid order of priority than they are now," Dr. Brick says. "Nowadays, if I think a patient might benefit from this drug early on, I'll explain the risks and benefits of methotrexate, compared with those of gold, and let the patient decide which she wants to try."

Q: What are the risks and benefits of methotrexate, compared with gold injections?

A: Both these drugs have potentially serious—even fatal —side effects, and require careful monitoring. Gold injections, for instance, may on rare occasions cause a potentially fatal allergic reaction called anaphylactic shock. Methotrexate can cause unexpectedly severe and sometimes fatal bone-marrow suppression and gastrointestinal toxicity, usually in people who are taking steroid drugs at the same time.

Gold is more likely than methotrexate to cause kidney damage; but methotrexate is more likely than gold to cause liver damage. Gold, not methotrexate, is likely to be prescribed to heavy drinkers.

Both drugs can cause serious changes in the blood that may require stopping its use, and both can cause birth defects. Both, too, have an array of bothersome side effects, such as skin rashes, nausea, loss of appetite and headaches.

Gold begins to work more slowly than methotrexate. People taking gold may begin to see improvement only after three to six months of treatment; people taking methotrexate may see improvement in one to two months.

About 80 percent of the people taking injected gold see an improvement in symptoms, but about one-third of them have to stop taking gold at some point because of side effects.

About 80 percent of the people taking methotrexate respond initially. And about 50 percent of people are still taking the drug with no problems five years after they start.

Stopping either drug can lead to a flare-up.

Because gold has been used so much longer than methotrexate, there are no surprises about its risks and benefits, including its possible long-term effects. With methotrexate, that's not the case. Many doctors say we won't know this drug's real benefits—or risks—for another 10 years or more.

And before you have to ask: Methotrexate treatment costs about $12 a week; injectable gold, about $47 a week (including the cost to get the injection); and oral gold costs $12.66 a week.

Q: How effective is methotrexate?

A: Studies show that about half of the people who take methotrexate get significant relief from their joint pain and swelling.

Q: How is methotrexate given?

A: Usually, it's given in pill form about once every 10 days. Sometimes it's given in weekly injections. And, as we already mentioned, methotrexate seems to kick in faster than gold: Benefits are seen in one to two months.

Q: How long do I have to take this drug?

A: Like other arthritis drugs, this is a long-term treatment. People may improve steadily over successive months, but if they stop taking the drug, they're likely to have a major flare-up within a few weeks. Some people have now been taking methotrexate for 10 years or longer with no serious side effects. (About 50 percent of people are still taking the drug with no problems five years after they first start.) But some researchers say it will take another 10 to 20 years before we know for sure just how safe—or dangerous—this drug really is.

Q: What kind of side effects do you need to watch out for with this drug?

A: The most common side effect is nausea, and that can be minimized by spreading your dose out over the day you take it. More troubling side effects include the suppression of new blood cells, which can lead to a severe form of **anemia**. For that reason, you must have regular blood tests while on this drug. Some doctors also give their patients a B-complex vitamin, folic acid, to reduce this side effect.

Liver damage is also possible with methotrexate, although doctors are finding that liver damage occurs less frequently than they'd anticipated. When used in large doses for the treatment of cancer, this drug has a high rate of liver damage. "About 1 out of every 100 to 200 people taking methotrexate for rheumatoid arthritis eventually develops some liver damage," says Dr. Grayzel of the Arthritis Foundation. "Liver damage appears to be much less common than we originally thought it would be, and it's not clear if people need to stop the drug if some slight liver damage appears. We don't know yet if they get worse if they continue on the drug."

Q: How do I find out if I have liver damage?

A: To check for liver damage, you need a blood test called a liver-chemistry profile every few weeks. A problem, though, is that severe liver damage may not show up on this blood test, so after two to three years of taking methotrexate, you may want to have a **liver biopsy** to make sure this vital organ is still in tip-top shape. Most doctors, however, do not require—or even offer—this test for their patients taking methotrexate, Dr. Grayzel says. They feel it's not necessary.

A liver biopsy is a relatively easy procedure. It's done in a hospital by a surgeon. After a local anesthetic is used to numb the skin, a hollow-core needle is inserted briefly into the liver, and a bit of the organ is removed. It does have a very small risk of fatal hemorrhage—less than 1 percent, according to Dr. Grayzel.

Q: **Sounds like I probably shouldn't be drinking alcohol if I'm taking this drug. Right?**

A: You're better off if you don't. In fact, you can help minimize the side effects of many drugs by avoiding more than an occasional drink. It's important to discuss with your doctor how much you actually do drink.

Q: **Are there other drugs I should know about?**

A: There are others, but they are used much less frequently than those we've mentioned and are not as well studied. They include azathioprine, chlorambucil and cyclophosphamide. Like methotrexate, these drugs suppress immune-system function.

Q: **So what other questions do I need to ask my doctor about the drugs he is prescribing?**

A: Any time you're handed a prescription, be prepared to ask questions. What is the exact name of this drug? For what condition or symptoms are you prescribing it? What it the drug supposed to do? How am I supposed to take it? Will it interact with any other drugs I am currently taking? (Refresh your doctor's memory if necessary. And include over-the-counter drugs.) What are the most common side effects? What are the most serious side effects? Should I stop the drug if I have side effects? How long will I be taking this drug? Is there any drug that has the same beneficial effects with fewer side effects?

Q: Is it safe to take a new drug that's been on the market only a short time?

A: "It's a good idea to wait until the drug has been out on the market for two or three years," Dr. Sack says.

Q: Why is that?

A: Because sometimes potentially dangerous side effects don't show up until a drug hits the market, Dr. Sack explains.

"As strict as the FDA is about allowing a drug on the market, and as well done as the studies may be, by the time a drug is marketed, at best only a few hundred people have taken it, and usually they are pretty healthy people. Then suddenly, 10,000 people start taking a drug. If a side effect, even a serious one, is only 1 percent, it might have escaped notice in the pre-marketing trials. All of a sudden, it's a major health hazard. A few hundred people are having liver failure or bleeding, or something like that."

SURGERY

Q: Is surgery ever used to treat arthritis?

A: Yes. Surgery may be done on a joint to reduce pain and improve function. And in some cases, it appears to slow the process of joint deterioration, at least for a time.

Q: What kinds of surgery are done?

A: Surgery can be done to trim back invading synovial tissue in a joint, to flush particles of debris out of a joint capsule, to smooth out rough cartilage, to improve the angle of impact on an eroding, lopsided knee, to immobilize painful, unstable joints, even to replace a joint that's become unbearably painful and useless.

Q: How long does a person stay on drug treatment before his doctor decides that surgery is needed to alleviate symptoms or restore function to a joint?

A: There is no definite answer. It varies from person to person. Let's just say that surgery is not usually the first line of treatment for any kind of arthritis—drugs are— but it's not necessarily a last resort either. The amount of time you give drug treatments or steroid injections before you move on to surgical options depends on many variables —which joints are affected, how badly damaged they are, the kind of surgery being contemplated, your general state of health, and others.

Some kinds of surgery prolong the life of a joint enough that you never require the ultimate in arthritis surgery—total joint replacement. "The right procedure, done for the right reasons, usually produces good results," says Steven Haas, M.D., a specialist in hip and knee-joint replacement surgery at the Hospital for Special Surgery in New York City.

Q: How can I determine if I would benefit from surgery?

A: If you have a painful joint that is no longer re- sponding to nonsurgical treatments, such as drugs, rest or steroid injections, your doctor should refer you to an orthopedic surgeon, also sometimes called a orthopedist.

Perhaps, too, you have certain problems in a joint, revealed by an x-ray or other imaging technique, that can be improved with surgery. If you have, for example, a severely overgrown synovium, bowed knees or other joint-alignment problems that are wearing down cartilage on one side of a knee, or intermittent pain in a knee that could be due to loose bits of cartilage in the joint capsule, your doctor may refer you to an orthopedic surgeon for possible surgery.

Q: What's the orthopedist going to do?

A: The orthopedic surgeon will examine your joints, look at your x-rays and probably take some of his own, and determine if indeed you would benefit from some kind of surgery. Your x-rays, for instance, may show that your hip-joint socket is pitted and that the shock-absorbing cartilage on the head of your thighbone is practically gone.

Q: Just because this surgeon finds a problem that surgery has been known to improve, does that mean I have to go through with it?

A: Of course not. Even after they've been told they could benefit from surgery, most people with arthritis have some time to explore their options, get a second opinion and find the best surgeon and hospital.

Furthermore, a person may be monitored closely for a while before any definite decisions are made regarding surgery. You see, some doctors, such as rheumatologists at large medical centers, work in groups that include orthopedic surgeons. If you're the patient of such a doctor, you may see an orthopedic surgeon early on for an evaluation; then you might see her every year or so for a reevaluation. Regular consultation with an orthopedist is one way to determine if or when surgery would be beneficial.

Q: What did you mean before by "the best surgeon and hospital"?

A: Anytime you go "under the knife," and in many cases under anesthesia, you want to have the most experienced and qualified surgeon you can find.

"Joint surgery, especially total joint replacement, is a highly technical operation, not just for the surgeon but for the whole surgical team, including the anesthesiologist," Dr. Haas says.

That means the best place for your operation is a hospital that performs your recommended surgery with great frequency, and the best doctor is one who does that procedure at least several times a week. It means that even if a doctor in your town says he can do and has done your surgery, you may want to compare his qualifications and frequency record with those of a medical team you'd get at a major university hospital in your region, preferably a National Institute of Arthritis and Musculoskeletal and Skin Diseases Multipurpose Center (see page 170 for a list of these).

Q: What kinds of surgery are available to people with arthritis?

A: One of the more common surgical procedures for people with rheumatoid arthritis is synovectomy. This is the surgical removal of some of the synovium, the lining of the fluid-filled capsule that surrounds a joint. A normal synovium is paper-thin in width. In a joint affected by rheumatoid arthritis, however, the synovium becomes inflamed and grows wildly, invading the joint capsule and eventually destroying cartilage and bone.

Synovectomy can be done on knees, wrists and fingers, but it is not done on hips.

Q: How does a surgeon work inside a joint capsule? Does he have to slice your whole joint open?

A: Not necessarily. For a knee joint, a doctor can use arthroscopic surgery.

Q: Arthroscopic surgery? What's that?

A: Arthroscopic surgery is surgery done on a joint using an **arthroscope**, a flexible viewing tube about the diameter of a pencil. The tube contains optical fibers, a small lens and a light scope. Inserted through a small incision into the joint capsule, an arthroscope provides the surgeon with a view of the joint's inside. The view can be magnified and displayed on a video screen. Instruments that fold down as they are passed through a channel in the arthroscope enable the surgeon to perform some procedures that formerly necessitated opening up the joint. The procedure is usually performed using a general anesthesia, but sometimes a spinal anesthesia is used. Arthroscopic surgery substantially reduces the time a patient needs to stay in the hospital.

Q: How is synovectomy done using arthroscopic surgery?

A: The joint capsule is distended by injecting air or fluid; the viewing tube is inserted through a small incision in the knee joint on one side, and a "cutting sweeper"—a tiny rotary blade attached to a suction tube—is inserted into the knee through two or three other small incisions. Using the viewing scope to guide him, the doctor maneuvers the cutting sweeper to slice off and suck out some of the overgrown synovial tissue.

Q: How is synovectomy done on other joints?

A: When it's done on smaller joints, such as the wrists or fingers, a synovectomy is done with an incision that exposes the synovium.

Q: What people most commonly have synovectomies?

A: Synovectomy is normally done only on people with a significant amount of inflamed tissue but little joint damage and it's done early in the course of the disease. "This surgery is indicated for someone whose inflamed joint has not improved with drugs or steroid injections, but whose x-rays still show healthy cartilage," Dr. Haas says.

Removing the synovium does not cure the underlying disease, but it can prevent a recurrence of inflammation in that joint, sometimes for a few years and sometimes permanently, according to Dr. Haas.

Q: Okay, so that's what a synovectomy is and does. What's another common surgical procedure for arthritis?

A: Arthroscopic debridement is a relatively common procedure, used only on knees. It flushes out of the joint capsule tiny bits of cartilage and bone, along with tissue-eroding enzymes. Any frayed edges of cartilage are removed at the same time, Dr. Haas says.

"Arthroscopic debridement is often done on people with osteoarthritis whose x-rays don't look too bad, yet they seem to get episodes of notable pain," Dr. Haas says. "They don't seem to be able to get by on anti-inflammatory drugs or steroid injections, but their joint is not bad enough for joint-replacement surgery." People with knees that lock up or catch because bits of cartilage are interfering with normal joint motion may see the best results from this surgery, he says.

Q: How well does this procedure work?

A: Sixty to 80 percent of people who have arthroscopic debridement on a knee have reduced pain for months and sometimes for as long as a year or so, Dr. Haas says. "There's currently no proof that this procedure does anything to slow the progress of the disease—that's something we want to study—but it entails little risk and quick recovery. Most people can walk out of the operating room."

Q: **Is arthroscopic surgery used for any other kinds of procedures?**

A: Yes. It can be used for a variety of joint "housekeeping and repair" chores, including cartilage and ligament repairs, pinning fractures in a joint and removing scar tissue.

Q: **Is arthroscopic surgery risky?**

A: Studies show it has an overall complication rate of about one-half of 1 percent. Risks include infection, nerve or blood-vessel damage and blood clots. As with any surgical procedure, it's best to find a doctor who does this type of surgery regularly.

Q: **Are there any other surgical techniques for the arthritic knee?**

A: Yes. One procedure, called an osteotomy, is performed to correct the angles at which the bones of a joint meet and, thus, to restore normal anatomy to an arthritic joint. It's most often done on knees. A wedge-shaped piece of bone is removed from above or below the joint to correct a bowleg or knock-knee and distribute the body's weight more evenly across the cartilage of the joint.

"Generally successful, this surgery is most often done on younger, active people with 'unicompartmental' osteoarthritis —arthritis on only one side of a joint," Dr. Haas says. It buys time for a joint in someone too young for an artificial joint, and may save a joint from ever needing to be replaced.

Q: **I've heard that people sometimes have joints fused to stop their pain. What's that procedure?**

A: The medicalese word for bone fusion is **arthrodesis.** In this surgical procedure, two or more bones in a diseased joint are joined together to prevent the joint from moving.

The precise technique used depends on which joint is being fused, but in most cases cartilage and a surface layer of bone are removed from each bone. The ends of the bones are then joined so that, when fresh bone cells grow, the ends fuse. The bones may need to be fastened in position with plates, rods or screws to immobilize the joint while the bones grow together. And sometimes a joint, such as a knee, may need to be immobilized for a time with pins inserted through the skin into the joint, to keep the joint from moving when body weight is applied. It can take up to six months for a fused joint to heal.

Q: **In what circumstances is this procedure done?**

A: Fusion is done when no other better options, such as joint replacement, are available, and treatments such as steroid injections have failed, Dr. Haas says. Fusing a joint generally does eliminate pain, and it can restore some function to a joint that had previously been useless, but it also reduces joint mobility to zero. If it's done on an ankle or knee, for instance, it affects the patient's gait. It's most likely to be done on wrists or ankles—there's no good replacement parts for those complicated joints—but it can also be done on knees, hips, ankles and fingers.

Q: **Do people with arthritis ever have bones removed? What's that procedure and when is it done?**

A: This surgery is called a resection. It involves removal of part or all of a damaged bone to help realign a joint that is permanently and painfully dislocated.

Resection can be done on any small joint, but it's done most frequently in the feet when damaged bones make walking painful in spite of treatment with drugs, steroid injections or orthopedic shoe inserts. Parts of the metatarsal bones, the long bones that extend from the ankles to the toes, are most likely to be removed.

A foot may be wider and flatter after this surgery, but the patient can still walk on it, often without pain. Resection may also be done to certain sections of the wrist or thumb.

Q: **You've mentioned joint replacement a couple of times. What is it?**

A: Joint-replacement surgery is a procedure to replace all or part of a joint—that is, the joining bones. A total-joint replacement, of course, replaces the whole joint.

Joint-replacement surgery is done when cartilage and underlying bone in a joint are so eroded and damaged that the joint hurts most of the time and the pain is severely limiting someone's activity.

Even though joint replacement often relieves pain and restores some function to joints, it's considered a last resort— an option to consider when drugs, steroid injections, rest and even less drastic forms of surgery have failed.

Q: **If it works so well, why would it be considered a last resort?**

A: All artificial joints have a limited life span, usually because they loosen or break. That life span is slowly increasing, though, thanks to better surgical techniques and more resilient replacement materials.

Q: **How long can I expect my artificial joint to last?**

A: That's something that varies from person to person, depending on his age, activity level and weight, among other things. The first generation of hip-joint replacements (those put in from 1968-74) were plagued by problems. Infection rates were high, and loosening and breakage were not uncommon. Now the track record is much better. Studies show that 9 out of 10 people who get a hip-joint replacement at age 60 still have a functioning hip 10 years later. Fifteen years later, 80 to 85 percent still have a functioning hip.

Artificial hips that are placed in younger people actually have a shorter life span, Dr. Haas says. Among people ages 50 to 60, only 80 percent still have a functioning hip joint 10 years after it's first installed. "They simply wear them out," Dr. Haas says. And no one knows what percentage of these joints will still be functioning after 15 or 20 years. That's why some doctors say any joint replacement before age 60 needs to be carefully considered.

Artificial knees, too, had big problems early on. The track record of early hinge-shaped knee-joint replacements was dismal. One study showed that more than 40 percent failed, and about 11 percent became infected.

Today's artificial knee-joint design sticks closely to the structure of an actual knee joint, using both plastic and metal to form a joint that not only bends, as the hinge joint did, but that also slightly twists and turns, like the real thing. These joints, used in one form or another since the mid-1970s, appear to have a life span as good as or slightly better than artificial hips, Dr. Haas says. Nine out of 10 people who get a knee replacement at age 60 still have a functioning knee 10 years later.

Q: **What about people younger than age 50? Do they ever get artificial joints?**

A: If at all possible, joint replacement is avoided in people younger than age 50. That may not be possible if someone has severe rheumatoid arthritis or osteoarthritis and needs this surgery to be able to function. "If you do joint replacement in someone that young, you have to be honest with them and tell them you don't know how long it is going to last," Dr. Haas says. "There's a fair to good likelihood that at some point during that person's lifetime the joint will need to be redone." That procedure is called a **revision**.

Q: A revision? Would you explain that?

A: Certainly. A revision is an operation to repair or replace an artificial joint that has loosened, broken or become infected. A revision doesn't last as long as the original joint replacement. "We generally expect a revision to last at least five years," Dr. Haas says. And doctors don't like to have to do more than one revision on a joint, because with each succeeding revision, the life span of the joint becomes shorter. But "you do what you gotta do," Dr. Haas says.

Revision requires at least as much surgical skill as the original joint replacement, perhaps more, if the doctor has to contend with bone loss from the loosened prosthesis. Here again, specialists emphasize, your best results should come from a doctor who does this sort of surgery several times a week.

Q: Let's back up for a minute. What joints are most likely to be replaced?

A: Hips, for starters. About 130,000 total hip replacements are performed each year. Knee-joint replacement is becoming increasingly popular, too, as better designs become available. About 130,000 total-knee-joint replacements are done each year.

Joint-replacement surgery can also be done on fingers and, much less frequently (because the results aren't that good), on shoulders and elbows.

Q: What exactly is done in joint-replacement surgery?

A: Any kind of joint replacement—whether it's a hip, knee or even a finger—is complicated, technically demanding surgery that requires a full crew of experienced sailors, orthopedic surgeons say.

For a hip replacement, done under general anesthesia, the surgeon makes a large incision on the side of the hip. He pushes or cuts through the surrounding muscles to expose the hip joint. He dislocates the joint, popping the ball-shaped head of the femur (thighbone) out of its socket in the pelvis. He saws off the head of the femur, then uses an instrument called a reamer to make the socket large enough to hold the cup-shaped artificial socket. He inserts the artificial socket.

Then he uses a coarse file to cut a shaft in the femur, and inserts the stem of the ball part of the artificial joint into the bone. He may or may not use a grouting-type cement to hold the stem in place.

He places the ball in the socket and, where necessary, reattaches muscles to bones with wires. Other muscles and tendons are replaced and repaired, and finally the incision is closed.

Q: And how is this surgery done for knees?

A: With knees, also done under general anesthesia, the surgeon usually makes one long incision on the front of the joint. He cuts through the joint capsule and synovium, then pushes aside the kneecap (patella) to get at the joint.

Special surgical tools are used to carefully measure the joint and to cut, shape and drill both the femur and the tibia (the larger calf bone) so that they can accept the artificial joint. Both are screwed into place and are often cemented.

The bottom half of the knee joint is a metal plate with a slight depression in its center. The top half is a metal cap that fits over this rounded bone. The metal cap rests in the bottom plate. Part of the back of the kneecap is cut away to give a flat surface, then drilled to accept the kneecap part of the joint.

Since the same ligaments that hold a natural knee joint in place are needed to maintain an artificial knee joint, only knees with intact or surgically repaired ligaments are acceptable for joint-replacement surgery.

Q: What about fingers?

A: Done before surrounding support tissues, such as tendons, have deteriorated, joint-replacement surgery of fingers restores pain-free motion. At least, that's the opinion of Richard R. McCormack, M.D., specialist in hand surgery at the Hospital for Special Surgery in New York City, among others. Usually it's only the largest knuckles that are replaced, and then only in people with rheumatoid arthritis.

Q: **Do people with osteoarthritis ever have finger-joint-replacement surgery?**

A: People with osteoarthritis may have bone-spur bumps around their knuckles that make their joints appear swollen, but they seldom lose the ability to use their hands, so they don't require surgery.

Q: **Is it better to have hand surgery done as soon as possible?**

A: That depends. It is true that decisions to operate on hands are made differently than decisions to operate on hips or knees. "If you delay having surgery, there's a risk of tendon rupture before the surgery," Dr. McCormack says. "We like to do the surgery before tendons rupture, because the results are much better."

There's no good way, however, to tell if tendon rupture is imminent, Dr. McCormack says. "That's why we have what we call a six-month rule. If you've had pain in your hands or wrists for six months and it hasn't responded to drugs or steroid injections, your risk of tendon rupture goes way up. We want to operate before that happens."

Q: **What material is used for a finger joint?**

A: Replacement finger joints are made out of a silicone-rubber material. They are one piece, a stem on either end and a flexible hinged piece in the middle. The stems insert into the bones of your finger, but they're not fixed in place. In fact, they move slightly in and out as you bend your fingers.

Q: **What goes on with this surgery?**

A: This surgery can take several hours, depending on how many joints are replaced and on what else is done to the hand, Dr. McCormack says. A regional anesthesia is used. It numbs part of the arm as well as the hand and fingers. An incision is made to expose the joint; the ends of the two diseased bones in the joint are cut away, along with diseased cartilage. The artificial joint is inserted, and the tissue and underlying skin are sewn up. If you have this surgery, your knuckles will be bandaged and your arm will be held upward in a sling to minimize swelling. You won't be able to use your hands at all for about four days, and you'll have limited use for about six to eight weeks, while you undergo extensive physical therapy. Just about everyone regains normal use of their hands in two to three months, Dr. McCormack says.

Q: **Is cement always used to hold a joint replacement in place?**

A: There are some new replacement joints on the market that don't need to be cemented into the bones. These joints have a fiber mesh or beaded surface that invites bone to grow into the artificial joint and, so, secure it. Cemented joints tend to loosen as tissue grows between the cement and the bone. It's thought that the new fiber-mesh joints will be less likely than cemented joints to loosen over time.

Q: **So how long are we talking about?**

A: No one knows for sure yet just how long these new noncemented joints will last. Studies so far seem to show that on the cup, or socket, side of a hip joint, the non-cemented component is very effective. There have been no high rates of early failure and no significant problems at 5 or 10 years.

On the stem side, however, results have been mixed. "In the short term, one or two years after surgery, the non-cemented joint tends to do worse than the cemented, in that patients are more likely to have thigh pain than they would with a cemented joint," Dr. Haas explains.

Results of studies have led many doctors to use a non-cemented socket in most hip-joint replacements, no matter what a person's age, and often a noncemented stem, or ball joint, in people younger than age 65.

"We know we can get predictably good results using a cemented joint in someone age 65 or older," Dr. Haas says. "But in someone younger and more active, the results with the cemented joint aren't as good. So even though we don't have all the data we would like, we might suggest a non-cemented joint to a younger person with good bone quality, hoping that we will achieve bone growth into the replacement joint, which may be more stable for the long term."

Q: **What about knees? Are they cemented?**

A: Noncemented knees have not worked as well as hips, and many doctors have stopped using them, at least for now.

Q: **I've heard so much about all the unnecessary surgery that's done on people. Do I need to worry about having unnecessary surgery for arthritis?**

A: There's no evidence to suggest that orthopedic surgery, such as total hip replacement, is performed without good reason. Still, whenever you're considering surgery, it's wise to get a second opinion, perhaps from a rheumatologist, who can check to make sure you've given all nonsurgical alternatives a fair try.

Orthopedic surgeons see patients every day for consultations, and not all of the patients end up having surgery, Dr. McCormack says.

"Some people's hands look really bad but they are functional. These people can do everything they need to do with them and don't really need surgery," he explains. "I talk with these patients, explain their options and what can be done, and talk about the likely outcomes and the risks. They then have the information they need and can make a decision."

And remember, no matter what your doctor tells you, it's up to you to decide whether or not to have surgery. Many times, with arthritis, that's a decision you can sit on for a while, because joint deterioration tends to be slow but steady. Sometimes, however, your surgery will turn out better if it's done promptly. That would be the case, for instance, if you had inflamed tendons that could rupture.

Q: Where should I go for surgery?

A: As we said earlier, for major orthopedic surgery, such a total joint replacement, and even for joint-reconstruction surgery, such as you might have done in a wrist, you want to use physicians who have high volume and great experience. If your surgeon replaces only a few joints a year, you may have a higher likelihood of infection or poor fit.

Some people first pick a big city hospital with a large orthopedic department, then find a surgeon with operating privileges at that hospital to perform their surgery. If the hospital where your doctor operates does not do a high volume in your type of surgery, chances are the nurses and anesthesiologists don't have the kind of familiarity with the procedure they would if they were assisting with it every day. And some smaller hospitals don't stock all sizes or types of joints, which may mean you receive a joint with a less-than-perfect fit, some doctors say.

Q: Any other questions I need to ask?

A: Often, several kinds of surgical procedures are used together to repair a joint, especially a complicated joint like a wrist. So ask exactly what procedures the doctor is recommending and why. Find out, too, what you can expect as a result of the surgery. Reduced pain? More strength in your hand? Increased mobility? Decreased mobility? Are you going to be able to walk? Play tennis? Open a jar? Scratch your back? Pick up a dime? And how long should those results last?

Ask, too, how long your recovery may take and what it entails. Major orthopedic surgery is inevitably followed by physical rehabilitation, and you want to make sure you're up to the challenge.

Q: Anything else I need to know?

A: If you're having joint-replacement surgery, you should get into the best possible health you can beforehand. If you have any kind of infection, even an aching tooth, you should have it treated before your surgery. Otherwise, there's a risk that the infection could travel to your new joint.

If you're overweight, your doctor will want you to drop some pounds before you have hip or knee-joint-replacement surgery. That's because your extra weight puts stress on your joint and could make it heal slower and loosen sooner.

Good muscle tone is important, too, so if you're able to do so, continue your exercise program.

If you're taking certain drugs for your arthritis, you may need to discontinue them for a week or two before your surgery. Be sure to talk to your physician and surgeon about this. Anti-inflammatory drugs and fish-oil capsules can increase the amount of time it takes for your blood to clot, making bleeding more of a problem. And some drugs for rheumatoid arthritis (methotrexate is one) may prevent a surgical wound from healing and, therefore, may have to be stopped for a time.

4 ALTERNATIVE SOURCES OF HELP

Q: In addition to drugs and surgery, are there other kinds of help for arthritis?

A: Yes, there are many. People with arthritis can choose from an international smorgasbord of treatments—from Chinese **acupuncture** to Swedish massage—to ease their aches and pains. Medical care for arthritis often includes physical therapy, exercise classes, occupational therapy and the use of joint-protecting splints, pain-easing massage, whirlpools, paraffin wax dips, heat and cold treatments, and other hands-on therapies. Several good studies now show that regular exercise can ease pain and improve joint mobility in just about everyone with arthritis, no matter what their age or how long they've had arthritis. We'll talk more about these studies and how to find an exercise program that suits you, a little later.

Q: Sounds like a lot of these treatments are performed by nonmedical providers. Is that true?

A: Yes. Many people with arthritis seek alternative medical treatments, such as acupuncture, herbal remedies or special diets. In fact, experts estimate that people with arthritis spend an impressive amount of money—perhaps a billion dollars a year—on a long, long list of alternative or scientifically unproven remedies, from copper bracelets to **DMSO (dimethyl sulfoxide)** to mussel extracts. Since these remedies aren't *proven* to work, at least not by the kind of scientific standards most M.D.'s would like to see, it's up to you to figure out whether a particular remedy is worth trying and what its possible risks are. In this chapter we'll tell you the kinds of questions you need to ask to evaluate a non-traditional remedy.

Q: Aren't there some treatments that involve diet and nutrition?

A: Yes. Some of these "nonproven" treatments include dietary changes. In fact, there is some intriguing evidence that dietary additions or deletions can help some people with arthritis, either by eliminating a symptom-producing food or by altering the body's inflammatory response. If you're interested in making dietary changes, we'll tell you how to get started safely.

Q: Aren't there treatments that are really experimental—where I become a guinea pig?

A: Some people with arthritis do indeed decide to become medical guinea pigs. They enroll in a research study, called a clinical trial, that examines a treatment that may have promise but that has not been proven to work. Some of these studies are federally funded and conducted at the National Institute of Arthritis and Musculoskeletal and Skin Diseases (NIAMS) or at one of the multipurpose arthritis centers at research and teaching hospitals around the country (see page 170). Other studies are funded by drug companies and may also be conducted at these multipurpose arthritis centers. We'll talk about some of these experimental treatments and what you need to know if you're interested in enrolling in a clinical trial.

EXERCISE

Q: Whew—it sounds like I really should have a lot of information before I start any treatment program. Can you tell me more?

A: Let's start with exercise, which gets top ratings from patients and doctors alike when it comes to relieving arthritis symptoms. In the *Arthritis: What Works* survey, in which, you'll recall, the authors amassed the answers of more than 1,000 people with arthritis, an overwhelming majority of participants said they exercise regularly because of their arthritis, and fully 95 percent said it helped. A small number said they found exercise too painful to pursue. And 17 percent had been hurt at least once by inappropriate or overzealous workouts—a good reason to get guidance before you begin.

Q: How does exercise help arthritis?

A: For both rheumatoid arthritis and osteoarthritis, a properly designed, faithfully done exercise program can get you moving and keep you moving. It can improve muscle strength, build stamina and allow joints to move better, with less pain and swelling. It also may allow some people to cut back on anti-inflammatory drugs. And it can replace feelings of fatigue and depression with new energy and optimism.

Q: How can I find a properly designed exercise program?

A: Start with the doctor who is treating your arthritis. Ask for a referral to a physical therapist—a professional who employs physical means to restore mobility and relieve pain and who must have at least a bachelor's degree—and seek one who treats people with arthritis. Working in conjunction with your doctor, the physical therapist can set up a daily exercise program to keep your joints as mobile and healthy as possible, or to help you recover from joint surgery. The physical therapist can show you exactly how to do the exercises and advise you on how much to do and when to cut back and rest. If you need special equipment to exercise —a splint, cane or special shoes—the therapist can also advise you.

A physical therapist is also likely to be involved in some of the more pleasant treatments associated with arthritis— whirlpool baths, hot-wax treatments for hands, and massage.

You may also want to call your local branch of the Arthritis Foundation, usually listed in the white pages of your phone book. The Arthritis Foundation produces several booklets and exercise videotapes for people with arthritis, and sponsors water-exercise classes at community pools around the country. (And in case you're shivering at the thought, pool-water temperature must be at least a balmy 84° for this class!)

Q: It sounds like most people with arthritis can at least kick around in a pool. What other kinds of exercise can they do?

A: People with arthritis are steered away from pounding, bouncy or jerky exercises, such as high-impact aerobics, racquet sports or running. But most can safely do many things: walking, bicycling, swimming, yoga, even weight lifting. The trick is to get your doctor's okay and proper instruction before you start doing any of these activities, so you don't suffer start-up injuries that put you permanently on the sidelines.

Many people do range-of-motion exercises regularly to keep their joints flexible. These exercises take each joint in the body through its full range. A physical therapist can teach you these exercises. And the Arthritis Foundation has a videotape that demonstrates range-of-motion exercises.

HEAT AND COLD

Q: I love whirlpool baths and hot tubs. Do they do anything to help my arthritis?

A: You may be in luck. Many people with arthritis find that settling into a hot tub of water soothes every joint in their body. Some use that buoyant, muscle-relaxing opportunity to do their range-of-motion exercises. Others use the whirlpool jets to give themselves a water massage. Pleasant as these soaks are, however, most people with arthritis say they offer only temporary relief.

Q: What about other forms of heat? What do they do?

A: Heating pads, electric blankets, even dipping the hands in hot paraffin wax, can all ease the stiffness and pain in aching joints, at least temporarily. Again, it's the heat, which increases blood flow to an area, that does the trick. In fact, many people with arthritis loosen up their stiff joints a bit with some form of heat prior to exercising.

Q: I've often heard that applying cold helps. Does it?

A: Cold, which reduces blood flow to an area, seems to work well to reduce pain and is usually your best choice for a hot, inflamed joint or a joint or muscle that's been overworked.

Q: Are there any risks with heat or cold treatments?

A: Heat is not always appropriate and can even aggravate some symptoms. Your best bet is to learn how to use both heat and cold with the guidance of a physical therapist. For instance, experts say you should not apply heat to one area for more than 20 to 30 minutes. And don't apply cold to one area for more than 10 to 20 minutes. Don't use heat or cold if you have poor circulation or poor sensation in the area. Don't use heat on a joint that's just been rubbed with a heat-producing analgesic cream, such as Ben-Gay, because the combination can damage your skin.

Q: What is a **deep heat** treatment?

A: This therapy uses tissue-penetrating ultrasound waves to heat up small areas of the body. In fact, this is the only heat treatment that can penetrate beyond the surface layers of the skin to a joint. In the Arthritis Survey, 81 percent of the people who tried ultrasound said it helped ease their pain and stiffness. Like other heat treatments, though, ultrasound is not always appropriate and may aggravate inflamed joints. This treatment is given by a physical therapist.

Q: How about massage? Does it help?

A: Massage can help relax tense muscles and improve circulation, and certain types of massage can help move fluid out of a swollen limb. But massage directly applied to a painful, inflamed joint can be harmful. If you're interested in getting a massage, ask your doctor or physical therapist for a referral to a massage therapist who works regularly with people with arthritis.

OCCUPATIONAL THERAPIST

Q: What about health-care professionals like occupational therapists? How can they help?

A: An occupational therapist—who has a bachelor's degree from an approved program and whose primary goal is to restore a degree of functioning—can show you how to protect your joints, carry on the normal activities of life in the best ways possible, and recommend special aids that make it easier to do things like open a jar, reach a high object, or even turn a steering wheel in a car.

An occupational therapist can also devise splints that help keep joints in normal positions, and so prevent permanent joint deformities that are hard to correct by reconstructive surgery.

Q: You've mentioned splints before. What exactly does a splint do?

A: A splint—usually made of plastic that can be heated slightly then molded around a wrist or finger—can prevent weak muscles from being stretched and can support joints by substituting for weak muscles. It can be used to keep an inflamed joint in its least painful position and reduce the possibility of a permanent deformity.

Some people wear wrist splints to bed, for instance, so that their wrists don't get bent into painful positions during the night. Others may wear them while using their hands for repetitive motions.

These days, though, doctors don't like to keep joints totally immobilized for too long for fear they'll become too weak and stiff to move. You may get a recommendation to remove your splint daily and put your joint through range-of-motion exercises.

CHIROPRACTOR

Q: What about chiropractors? How are they trained? Can they help someone with arthritis?

A: A chiropractor is a nonmedical doctor who holds the degree of doctor of chiropractic care (D.C.) and is licensed to provide chiropractic treatments. These treatments involve spinal manipulation, or adjustments, in which the chiropractor pushes on the vertebrae to reposition them. Chiropractic is based on the principle that the spinal column is central to a person's entire sense of well-being because it is instrumental in maintaining the health of the nervous stem. Through chiropractic adjustments, the nervous stem is kept in or returned to good health.

Since chiropractors are concerned with the structure of the body, they are required to study anatomy, physiology, neurophysiology, biomechanics and kinesiology. This training, as well as the use of certain diagnostic procedures, permits chiropractors to consider the body's entire neuro-musculoskeletal system when making a diagnosis.

Chiropractic adjustments may offer people with arthritis some temporary relief, the Arthritis Survey found. That relief may come in the form of increased mobility in a stiffened spine, says Scott Haldeman, M.D., D.C., Ph.D., associate clinical professor in the department of neurology at the University of California at Irvine.

But overall, this survey gave chiropractors the lowest ratings of all widely seen practitioners—M.D. or non-M.D.—in part because a sizable percentage of people, 14 percent, felt worse after they'd seen a chiropractor.

"It's important to use nonforce mobilization techniques during acute inflammation," Dr. Scott explains. "Otherwise you may feel some temporary increase in pain." He suggests you tell your chiropractor if your symptoms have changed since his initial evaluation of you. You should also tell your chiropractor if you feel like you're having a flare-up.

PSYCHOLOGIST

Q: **What if I'm having trouble coping with my illness? Who can I see then?**

A: A **psychologist** may be able to help you adjust to your illness and limitations, if you have any, and to help you free up your mental energies so you can get on with your life. Some psychologists can also teach techniques such as biofeedback and progressive relaxation, that studies have shown do reduce pain and stress, so that you may require less medication, sleep better and feel more in control.

Shop for a psychologist as you would for any health-care professional. Ask the doctor treating your arthritis for a referral, and ask other people with arthritis. Call the local

Arthritis Foundation and ask for a referral to a psychologist who treats people with arthritis or other chronic illnesses.

Have a get-acquainted visit, and, based on your impressions from that first visit, decide if this psychologist is your best choice for help.

NUTRITIONIST

Q: **You mentioned earlier that nutrition and dietary changes may help some people with arthritis. What kind of health-care professional would I see for that?**

A: Either a **nutritionist** or **registered dietitian** can help you make dietary changes.

If you need to lose weight to take a load off aching knees, for instance, a nutritionist or dietitian can help you devise a weight-loss program that allows you to lose weight sensibly and gradually, without compromising good nutrition. Either one can also help you select vitamin and mineral supplements when appropriate, and steer you through the maze of dietary treatments for arthritis, which we'll discuss shortly.

Q: **What's the difference between a nutritionist and a dietitian?**

A: Anyone can call herself a nutritionist, whether or not she has special training in nutrition. On the other hand, only people who have been certified in dietetics by the American Dietetic Association (ADA) can call themselves registered dietitians (R.D. for short). It's sort of a trademark. No one else can use it.

According to the ADA, to be a registered dietitian a person must have a bachelor's degree in foods and nutrition or dietetics from an accredited college or university; complete a work-study program or internship (usually lasting 12 months or more and always ADA-approved) to gain practical experience; pass a national qualifying examination administered by the ADA; and maintain the R.D. status through continuing-education courses.

Q: Does this mean I should choose an R.D. for a nutritionist?

A: Not necessarily. They are sources of valid information from their perspective, but many authorities in the field contend that the R.D.'s perspective is outdated—too focused on the four basic food groups and food management rather than more timely issues, such as supplementation and preventive medicine.

So don't accept at face value any person's credentials without asking a lot of questions.

The American Nutritionists Association, P.O. Box 34030, Bethesda, MD 20817, can provide you with a list of nutrition consultants in your area, all of whom have advanced degrees in nutrition from reputable schools. The ANA asks that you enclose a self-addressed stamped envelope and $1, and stipulate which state list you want.

You can get a list of registered dietitians by sending a self-addressed stamped envelope and $1 to the American Dietetic Association, 430 N. Michigan Ave., Chicago, IL 60611.

Q: Are there any alternative treatments I should avoid?

A: It all depends. It's always wise to approach any new treatment—even popular arthritis drugs—with skepticism, to find a practitioner with lots of experience, and, if you're using a treatment at home, to make sure you really do know how to do it and its potential hazards. Even something as simple as a heating pad can do harm if used the wrong way.

Ask questions to determine if the treatment is appropriate and helpful for your condition. Are there any studies published that show its effectiveness for arthritis? What has been the practitioner's experience in using the treatment for arthritis? Can you talk with other arthritis patients who have used the treatment? Do you feel better after you've had a treatment?

To return to the Arthritis Survey—some 14 percent of the people who saw a chiropractor said they felt worse after treatment. That percentage was the highest for any practitioner in the survey. And 17 percent of the surveyed people said that they'd been hurt at least once by inappropriate or overzealous exercise.

DIET

Q: I've heard that certain foods can cause arthritis, or at least make it worse. Is that true?

A: Only one type of arthritis, gout, has been definitely connected with diet. Foods high in **purines**—protein compounds found in anchovies, organ meats and mushrooms, among other foods—can aggravate the condition by elevating body levels of uric acid. The uric acid builds up to high levels in synovial fluid and forms joint-irritating crystals.

Some intriguing research findings, however, do suggest that food plays a role in other types of arthritis as well, or at least in some sorts of joint inflammation that may resemble arthritis. Food may provoke joint inflammation in two ways, which we'll detail a bit later. Meanwhile, here are some suggested links between food and arthritis.

In a small number of sensitive people, certain foods may provoke an allergic inflammatory reaction in joint tissue, just as it might cause hives or asthma in other sensitive people. So they may find that eliminating these foods from their diets helps relieve joint inflammation.

The kinds of fat a person eats seem to influence the body's inflammatory response, too. Researchers believe that some fats promote the manufacture of inflammation-producing biochemicals, while other fats, such as fish oil, interfere with the manufacture of inflammation-producing biochemicals. Indeed, some studies show that certain fatty acids can be helpful to people with rheumatoid arthritis.

Q: Wait—let's talk about food allergies and arthritis. What kind of studies have been done? What do they show?

A: The food-arthritis link is highly controversial, and most doctors believe there are not enough hard facts (i.e., good, controlled clinical studies) to say for sure that food sensitivities can cause arthritis, especially when it comes to rheumatoid arthritis.

"That a food might cause symptoms of arthritis is a scientific theory, not a fact. That means it's not proven," points out Richard S. Panush, M.D., professor and chairman of the department of medicine at St. Barnabas Medical Center in Livingston, New Jersey, and a leading researcher in this area. (You may recall from chapter 2 that the cause of rheumatoid arthritis remains unknown, although many suspect it starts with exposure to something that alters immune response—perhaps a virus or bacteria.)

Research into the food-arthritis link includes single case studies (in which a doctor looks at one patient), a few animal studies and a few dietary-restriction studies (in which people with rheumatoid arthritis tried a certain kind of diet to see if their symptoms improved).

Several of the single case studies were done by Dr. Panush, as he puts it, "to prove once and for all" that there is no truth to the common belief that food has anything to do with arthritis. His studies seem to indicate, instead, that a small number of people do indeed get flare-ups of arthritis when they eat certain foods.

Q: What more can you tell me about these case studies?

A: So far Dr. Panush has tested 15 people who believe that certain foods aggravate their joint pain. Of those 15, 10 showed no reaction to food, two had mixed responses, and three experienced arthritis symptoms when given food disguised in capsules. One reacted to milk, another to shrimp, and the third to **nitrates**, a common food preservative.

The first person Dr. Panush tested was a 52-year-old woman who insisted her arthritis was caused by meat, milk and beans. She agreed to go on an extremely restricted diet for several weeks and ate nothing except a liquid diet food called Vivonex. The result was that she was not bothered by stiff joints during this time.

Then, in what's called a double-blind, placebo-controlled manner, she was given the foods she claimed were causing her symptoms. In this tightly controlled test, neither she nor the people giving her the foods knew what foods she was receiving. The foods, in powdered form, were in opaque capsules. And not all the capsules contained a food she claimed were causing her symptoms. Some were placebos— harmless sugar pills.

At the end of this study, it was clear that the culprit was milk. When the woman ate capsules of powdered milk, her morning stiffness and tender, swollen joints returned. Symptoms were worst within 24 to 48 hours after ingesting the milk, and subsided within three days. The milk dosage in the capsules was comparable to one eight-ounce glass of milk per meal.

Q: Okay, so milk may be a problem for some people. Are there other foods that cause symptoms of arthritis?

A: In individual case reports by other researchers, cheese, corn, wheat and other foods have been associated with RA-like symptoms.

Q: What about animal studies?

A: In a study with rabbits, rheumatoid-like inflammation of the synovium, the tissue lining the inside of the joint capsule, was induced simply by substituting cow's milk for water in the diet.

Q: And dietary-restriction studies?

A: Several studies have looked at all sorts of dietary restrictions. The results of these studies have been mixed.
Dr. Panush, for instance, tested a popular arthritis diet, called the Dong diet after the doctor who invented it, Collin H. Dong, M.D. The diet eliminated red meat, additives, preservatives, fruit, dairy products, herbs, spices and alcohol. The diet improved symptoms in a few people but seemed to work no better than a diet that arbitrarily eliminated foods like sour cream, turkey, bananas and cornflakes, while allowing red meat and white wine. Dr. Panush noted that a few people did seem to exhibit reduced joint swelling on the Dong diet. Some of those people were later tested individually, and a few were found to be sensitive to certain foods.

Q: I've heard that a vegetarian diet can help people with arthritis. Does it? How does it work?

A: Yes, it has been noted that people with rheumatoid arthritis do better on a vegetarian diet. However, only one study, by researcher Lars Skoldstam of the Sundvalls Hospital, in Sundvalls, Sweden, has looked at the effects of a vegetarian diet on rheumatoid arthritis. In that study, 60 percent of the people with rheumatoid arthritis who followed a **vegan diet**—which excludes meat and dairy products—said they felt better on the diet. We should mention, too, that the diet also excluded or limited use of refined sugar, corn, flour, salt, strong spices, alcohol, tea and coffee.

This researcher didn't claim to know how the diet worked, but it's possible it eliminated some of the foods to which people with rheumatoid arthritis were sensitive. In the Arthritis Survey, foods people said they were most likely to avoid included red meat, sugar, fats, salt, caffeine and alcohol.

Q: What about not eating at all?

A: Yes, **fasting**—going without food—does seem to relieve symptoms in people with rheumatoid arthritis, according to several studies. Unfortunately, in most cases, the relief disappears soon after the fast is broken.

In one Swedish study, 8 out of 10 people said they felt much better while fasting. For 11 days, they had nothing but vegetarian broths, juices made from vegetables or berries and herbal teas every two or three hours. We should mention, however, that two members of the group grew worse.

Q: What is it about fasting that relieves symptoms of arthritis in some people?

A: Fasting has a modulating effect on the immune system, according to other researchers. It slows the action of certain enzymes and blocks the production of biochemicals that cause inflammation.

Other researchers point out that fasting eliminates any symptom-causing foods. Some think it may improve conditions in the bowel, at least temporarily. Some forms of inflammatory arthritis have been associated with inflammatory bowel disease.

If you're in good health and not taking drugs, most doctors agree that one to three days of fasting won't hurt you. But most people with RA don't fit that bill. They're underweight and may even be malnourished. For them, the risks of fasting could outweigh its short-term benefits.

Q: Alright, we've established that, for some people, food might be a factor in joint pain. But what's the mechanism behind it?

A: The mechanism has to do with the body's immune system. In cases in which a food seems to be causing an allergic reaction, researchers speculate that it works like this: Somehow a person's intestinal wall becomes permeable

—meaning it allows passage of things that would normally be blocked. This may be due to inflammation, bacterial overgrowth, an allergic tendency or even taking anti-inflammatory drugs. The intestinal wall allows large molecules of a food—milk, for instance—that it doesn't normally allow, to pass through the intestinal membrane and into the bloodstream. There, the molecules of milk are treated by the body's immune system as though they were harmful invaders, such as bacteria or viruses, explains Terry Phillips, Ph.D., director of the immunogenetics and immunochemistry laboratory at George Washington University Medical Center, in Washington, D.C.

In response to the milk molecules (called antigens), the body's immune cells develop antibodies. The antibodies can do a number of things, Dr. Phillips explains: "They can latch onto the milk antigen as it's absorbed through the gut, and become a creature called a circulating immune complex, which goes around in the body's bloodstream until it can find a good place to be deposited. Circulating immune complexes may stick to blood-vessel walls, where they cause hives and vasculitis. Or a very common place for them to go is into the joints, especially if the joint is already damaged by an arthritic flare-up." In the joint, the immune complexes lie on the synovium, the tissue lining the joint capsule. There, they attract what Dr. Phillips calls the "garbage-collection cells," macrophages, which gobble up the immune complexes and tear up the joint tissue as well, causing localized inflammation.

It's also possible for a food antigen to travel alone to a joint, and there, be attacked by antibodies that are on the surface of **mast cells** in the synovium. When this happens, the mast cells detonate like microscopic bombs, releasing a spray of inflammatory biochemicals into your joint that destroys the milk antigen and perhaps damages a few joint cells as well.

A similar allergic response can occur in almost any organ in the body, says Dean Metcalfe, M.D., head of the mast-cell physiology section of the National Institutes of Allergy and Infectious Disease, in Bethesda, Maryland. "A person's genetic predisposition may determine which organs are targeted for an allergic response."

Q: What percentage of people with rheumatoid arthritis have symptoms aggravated by food?

A: The official figure (i.e., the one that seems to be most accepted) is 5 percent or less, according to Dr. Panush. But some doctors claim, without hard evidence to prove it, that the figure may be as high as 30 percent.

Dr. Panush notes that people whose arthritis is affected by food do not show some of the other classic symptoms of rheumatoid arthritis, such as joint deterioration and the presence of rheumatoid factor in the blood. In fact, he likes to call food-aggravated arthritis *allergic arthritis* to distinguish it from rheumatoid arthritis.

Q: Do people with rheumatoid-arthritis pain have many allergic symptoms, such as skin or nasal allergies?

A: Research seems to indicate that they do not, says Dr. Metcalfe. "Allergic disease is no more common in people with RA than it is in the general population, and people with allergies are not particularly prone to RA."

Q: What foods are most likely to cause symptoms of arthritis?

A: As we said earlier, research is scant, but in several studies milk or cheese was found to cause symptoms. In fact, researchers in Switzerland have found changes in the immune system of people who appear to be milk-sensitive. Those same researchers tested two people who appeared to be highly sensitive to whole milk and found they reacted to a specific protein in milk. Corn, shrimp, nitrates, beef and wheat have also been implicated in some cases.

Some researchers believe, too, that a certain family of vegetables, called **nightshades**, can cause symptoms of joint inflammation for some people.

Q: What are nightshades?

A: Nightshades are a botanical family that includes potatoes, eggplants, tomatoes and peppers (red and green bell peppers, chili peppers and paprika, but not black pepper). This group also includes tobacco and some other very toxic plants, such as belladonna (called *deadly night-shade*), henbane, mandrake and jimsonweed.

Even the edible members of this family have long been viewed with suspicion. As recently as the early 1800s most Americans and Europeans thought raw tomatoes could kill you.

Q: But can they cause arthritis?

A: Andrew Weil, M.D., professor of medicine at the University of Arizona College of Medicine and author of several books on alternative medicine, including *Natural Health, Natural Medicine* (Boston: Houghton Mifflin, 1990) says this: "Some medical practitioners do warn their arthritis patients away from them. Actually a small percentage of arthritis sufferers are nightshade sensitive and will experience benefit if they eliminate all foods containing these vegetables."

The doctor who came up with the no-nightshades diet, Norman F. Childers, Ph.D., a now-retired Rutgers University horticulture professor, believes a number of substances, including **solanine**, that are found in all these plants cause symptoms. Solanine is a known toxin, and in animals it has been associated with joint inflammation. However, most doctors believe you don't get enough of it in any of these foods to do you harm.

Dr. Childers says he has surveyed thousands of people with arthritis who tried his no-nightshade diet, and says about 70 percent say they find some relief on this diet.

Q: If I want to try this diet, what should I do?

A: You should learn how to read food-package labels. Potato starch and tomato flakes or paste are found in many foods. Also, you should avoid tobacco for many reasons, not just to comply with this diet.

As we said earlier, the Arthritis Survey indicates that quite a few people avoid one food or another. Their collective list of foods to avoid included red meat, sugar, fats, salt, caffeine, nightshades (tomatoes, potatoes, pepper and eggplant), alcohol, junk foods, starches (such as wheat), citrus, pork, smoked or processed meats and dairy products. Of course, most people don't need to avoid all these foods but only one or a few. Figuring out which ones are off limits for you, though, takes some trying.

Q: How can I determine which foods, if any, are causing my symptoms?

A: One way is to start keeping a journal in which you record everything you eat and in which you also record and rate your joint pain and any swelling. If your symptoms vary from day to day, keeping a food journal might help you pinpoint troublesome foods.

Another way is to eliminate all forms of the suspected food from your diet for about two months, then add it back to your diet and see if your symptoms flare up.

Some foods, especially those you eat all the time or that are found in many different foods (wheat, for instance), can be difficult to connect with symptoms.

ALLERGIST

Q: You mean that if a food I eat frequently is causing my symptoms, I may not figure out what it is?

A: Yes, and you may find you need the help of an allergist who treats people with food sensitivities. Not all do, and some have much more experience with food-related symptoms than others. Some allergists have a special interest in what they call *environmental medicine*—the effect of environment, including foods, air and water, on people's health. These doctors refer to themselves as **environmental physicians**. They were formerly called clinical ecologists.

To find an allergist, ask your primary-care doctor for a referral, or contact either of these organizations for a referral: American Academy of Allergy and Immunology, 611 E. Wells St., Milwaukee, WI 53202; (414) 272-6071; or American Academy of Environmental Medicine, P.O. Box 16105, Denver, CO 80216; (303) 622-9755.

Q: What can an allergist do to help?

A: An allergist can devise a diet that allows you to avoid the offending food substance. Doctors use different sorts of diets. Some use a diet of foods so seldom eaten that someone is unlikely to have developed allergies to them. Those foods might include buckwheat, mangoes, pheasant, kiwi fruit and turnips, for instance. Another doctor might put you on a diet of lamb, pears and springwater.

After a period of time on this diet—a week, perhaps—you'll be asked to reintroduce a specific food and see if your symptoms worsen. If they do worsen, you may want to continue to avoid that food.

Of the 10 participants in the Arthritis Survey who saw an allergist or clinical ecologist, 7 said they'd been helped dramatically.

Q: You said earlier that fats in my diet can influence my body's inflammatory response. How does that work?

A: The type of fat you eat helps to determine, at least to some extent, your body's manufacture of hormone-like biochemicals called prostaglandins. Some prostaglandins promote inflammation; others inhibit inflammation. The fatty acids in foods are the precursors, or building blocks, for prostaglandins. Your body takes the fatty acids you eat and, through a series of metabolic steps, assembles them into either pro-inflammatory or anti-inflammatory prostaglandins.

Q: What kinds of fats are pro-inflammatory?

A: Most vegetable oils—safflower, sunflower, corn, sesame and soy oil—are rich in the class of fatty acids known as omega-6 fatty acids. These fatty acids create the inflammatory prostaglandin called leukotriene. (Aspirin and other NSAIDs work by blocking the formation of leukotriene.)

FISH OILS

Q: What kinds of fats are anti-inflammatory?

A: Two kinds seem to be anti-inflammatory: **omega-3 fatty acids** (also called **eicosapentaenoic acid,** or EPA) found in fatty fish; and **gamma-linolenic acid (GLA),** found in high concentrations in black-currant oil, evening-primrose oil and borage oil.

Q: I've heard a lot lately about fish oils. What are they?

A: Omega-3 fatty acids are oils that are found mostly in cold-water fatty fish like mackerel, sardines and salmon. They're also found in purslane, a fleshy weed that's easily grown in home vegetable gardens. Omega-3 fatty acids are liquid at room temperature and remain liquid even at very low temperatures.

You've probably heard about them in conjunction with heart disease. They have been found to reduce clotting tendency in blood and, so, to lower risk of heart attack. They've also been shown to inhibit inflammation, by interfering with the production of inflammatory biochemicals and altering certain aspects of the immune system.

Q: How do they help people with rheumatoid arthritis?

A: Six studies have been done so far that have examined the effects of omega-3 fatty acids on people with rheumatoid arthritis. All have shown a modest beneficial effect, reports Joel Kremer, M.D., professor at Albany Medical College, in New York, and a leading researcher in this field.

Dr. Kremer's most recent study, for instance, compared people with active RA who took high or low doses of omega-3 fish oils with those who took olive oil. Both the high- and low-fish-oil groups saw more of an improvement in symptoms than the olive-oil group saw. But the high-dose fish-oil group did best, improving in 21 of 45 clinical measures, including grip strength, number of swollen joints and the length of time they could remain active without becoming tired.

In the studies Dr. Kremer and others have done, the people who take fish oil also continue to take their arthritis medications. Improvement in symptoms usually is not seen until after at least 12 weeks of continuous use and appears to increase with extended treatment intervals of 18 to 24 weeks, Dr. Kremer says.

Doses have varied from study to study, and determining the ideal dosage and formulation, even whether fish oils "should be used as an occasional adjunct or as a replacement for certain components of the traditional RA drug regimen" remains to be determined, writes Dr. Kremer in a recent review article.

Q: What about that gamma acid you mentioned earlier?

A: Gamma-linolenic acid, also liquid at room temperature, is found in concentrated amounts in blackcurrant oil, evening-primrose oil and borage oil. It, too, seems to inhibit inflammation, by suppressing the production of biochemicals that cause inflammation. However, this oil has been studied less than the omega-3 fatty acids.

In a study at the Royal Infirmary in Glasgow, Scotland, doctors found that gamma-linolenic acid, alone or in combination with omega-3 fish oils, gave a number of people with mild rheumatoid arthritis enough pain relief to allow them to stop taking their nonsteroidal anti-inflammatory drugs.

One group of people in this study took 12 capsules a day of evening-primrose oil. Another group took a combination of fish oil and evening-primrose oil. A third group took a harmless look-alike capsule of paraffin.

At the end of three months, all the patients tried to cut down on their drugs, but were told to do so only if their symptoms did not worsen. Of the 28 patients who were able to stop or reduce their drugs, 11 were taking evening-primrose oil at the time, and 12 were taking the combination of fish oil and evening-primrose oil.

Q: So what's all this mean to me in terms of my diet?

A: Doctors who are incorporating these findings into their dietary recommendations for people with rheumatoid arthritis suggest this:

• Make sure you eat enough to maintain your normal body weight. That's something many people with RA fail to do, either because they're avoiding foods they think are causing symptoms, taking drugs that cause nausea or gastrointestinal upset, or have limited mobility that makes it hard for them to shop or cook.

• Make sure you are getting the Recommended Dietary Allowance (RDA) of every nutrient, which is hard to do even when you are active and are eating a high-calorie diet. You may want to take multivitamin-mineral and individual supplements as necessary. The RDA is the amount of a nutrient deemed adequate for preventing nutritional-deficiency-related diseases.

• Keep your total-fat intake fairly low, at about 25 percent of calories from fat. That means you should eat plenty of grains and vegetables and stick with lean cuts of meat and low-fat dairy foods.

• Reduce your intake of safflower, sunflower, corn, sesame or soy oil by cutting back on salad dressings, fried foods and margarine.

• Increase your intake of fish oil. The safest, easiest way to do this is by eating three meals a week of fatty fish. If you want to take fish-oil capsules, discuss dosage with your doctor.

Some doctors also recommend that you increase your intake of gamma-linolenic acid by taking capsules containing this oil. Gamma-linolenic acid does not occur in large amounts in any commonly eaten food, so it's hard to come by in most diets. Other doctors don't think there is enough research yet to make this recommendation.

Q: **Do I need medical supervision to make these dietary modifications?**

A: Some doctors say yes, others, no. We recommend you consult your doctor before you make any major changes in diet, including adding fish oils or gamma-linolenic acid. In studies so far, these oils seem to be safe. However, researchers point out that no one knows the possible risks associated with long-term, high-dose use of these oils.

VITAMINS AND MINERALS

Q: **What about vitamins and minerals? Do any in particular help arthritis?**

A: Here again, there's a real lack of solid research. But to answer your question, so far no one vitamin or mineral seems to stand out as having a significant impact on either rheumatoid arthritis or osteoarthritis.

In the Arthritis Survey, more than 70 percent of people said they take some vitamins, usually a one-a-day multivitamin, and about half of the vitamin takers found it helpful.

Some vitamins and minerals, such as calcium, selenium and vitamin C, are known to be involved in the formation of bone, cartilage and connective tissue, or in the formation of biochemicals that have anti-inflammatory properties in the body. And there is speculation that some play a role in rheumatoid arthritis, osteoarthritis or inflammation in general. These are all good reasons to make sure you are getting the RDA of every essential nutrient.

Q: **I've heard it's important for people with arthritis to take plenty of vitamin C. Is that true?**

A: It may well be. Inflammation tends to deplete the body's stores of vitamin C. Compounding the problem, nonsteroidal anti-inflammatory drugs interfere with vitamin C metabolism and excretion. Research also shows that people with rheumatoid arthritis have significantly lower blood levels of vitamin C than people without RA, irrespective of drug therapy. For these reasons, some doctors recommend higher-than-normal doses of vitamin C for their patients with RA. Dr. Weil, for instance, recommends 3,000 milligrams a day of vitamin C, 50 times the RDA. Research has shown that vitamin C is remarkably safe, even in large amounts.

In one study, British researchers who gave 500 mg. of vitamin C daily to people with rheumatoid arthritis found a dramatic lessening of the bruising frequently associated with RA. In another study, supplemental vitamin C perked up sluggish immune response in people with RA. Other studies, however, have found no effect on the course of rheumatoid arthritis, either with large daily doses or with injections of vitamin C directly into the joint.

Q: Are people with arthritis low in any other nutrients?

A: Yes, perhaps because they're so often malnourished, people with RA often have quite a few nutritional deficiencies.

A study by Finnish researchers showed reduced blood levels in people with RA for vitamins A and E, along with zinc. All three of these nutrients play a role in immune function and may help control inflammation in the body.

In one study, large doses of zinc (50 mg., three times a day) improved symptoms in 12 of 24 people with RA. These people had not responded well to other forms of treatment. In another study, zinc supplementation improved some symptoms in people with psoriatic arthritis (inflammatory arthritis coupled with the skin disease psoriasis). However, another study showed no improvement after zinc supplementation in people with long-standing RA.

Q: Do doctors make any recommendations about these nutrients?

A: Here again, some researchers suggest that rheumatoid-arthritis sufferers eat foods rich in vitamin E, zinc and beta-carotene (a plant substance converted to vitamin A in the body). Dr. Weil goes a step further. He recommends 25,000 international units a day of beta-carotene, and 400 I.U. of vitamin E (800 I.U. if you are over 40). Research shows both these nutrients to be quite safe, even in large amounts. Large amounts of zinc, however, can cause problems.

Q: Are people with RA low in other nutrients?

A: Yes. A study found that blood levels of pantothenic acid, a B-complex vitamin, were significantly lower in people with RA than in healthy people. Studies in animals have shown that young rats acutely deficient in pantothenic acid suffer defects in growth and development of bone and

cartilage. Two British studies looked at supplementation of pantothenic acid in people with RA. In both studies, supplementation led to some improvement in symptoms.

Selenium, a trace mineral involved in immune-system functioning—and which may act both as an anti-inflammatory and a pro-inflammatory—has also been found to be low in people with RA. Injected and oral selenium and vitamin E preparations are used, with reportedly good results, in veterinary practice to relieve arthritic inflammation in dogs and other animals. But there are no good studies of its use in people with RA. Dr. Weil recommends a daily 50 microgram supplement (a microgram is one-millionth of a gram) of selenium to people with RA. More is not better when it comes to selenium. Large amounts are toxic.

Vitamin B6 supplements are sometimes recommended to people with RA, especially if they suffer from carpal tunnel syndrome, a pinched nerve in the wrist, or tarsal tunnel syndrome, the same problem in the ankle. In several small studies, vitamin B6 reduced pain and symptoms of numbness in some people with carpal or tarsal tunnel syndrome. Large doses of vitamin B6 can cause nerve problems, however, and should be taken only with medical supervision.

Studies also indicate that people with RA have depressed iron levels and mild anemia, due in part to problems the body has using its stores of iron—probably because of disease. Usually, this anemia does not respond to iron therapy. Intravenous infusions of an iron-sugar solution in RA patients were observed to precipitate flare-ups, which has led some researchers to raise the possibility that excessive quantities of iron may be harmful in people with inflammatory diseases. So the use of iron supplementation in people with RA is controversial. Some doctors believe it should be avoided.

Q: What about copper—and copper bracelets?

A: The official word from the medical establishment on copper bracelets is "just plain silly." The Arthritis Survey participants who tried some sort of copper jewelry— 211 out of 1,051—didn't find it particularly helpful. Some 85 percent said it did nothing, 6 percent said it helped, and another 7 percent said it may have helped.

Only one study has been done that looks at copper bracelets and arthritis. In that Australian study, 240 "arthritis/
rheumatism" sufferers were randomly assigned to one of
three groups. Group I wore a copper bracelet for one month
followed by a placebo bracelet (aluminum) for one month.
Group II wore the two bracelets in reverse order, while
group III wore no bracelets at all. Of the 77 people who
completed the study, 47 noted a difference between the
bracelets. Some 37 of the 47 perceived the copper to be more
effective. These researchers also found that copper bracelets
lose weight after they're worn for a while, which may mean
that copper is being absorbed from the bracelet into the body.

So the bottom line is this: Wear one if you want, but don't
count on it to relieve your symptoms. And by all means,
don't abandon other treatments that do work.

Q: What about copper in my diet? Is it important?

A: Copper is thought to play a role in rheumatoid
arthritis. Just what that role might be isn't understood. Researchers know that copper levels are elevated in
both the blood and synovial fluid of people with RA, but
they don't know if that means the body is mobilizing copper
stores to fight inflammation.

Q: What else is known?

A: In his book *The Doctor's Vitamin and Mineral
Encyclopedia* (New York: Simon and Schuster, 1990),
Sheldon Saul Hendler, M.D., Ph.D., says copper is known to
be involved in the production of several proteins, including
collagen and elastin. Collagen is responsible for the functional integrity of bone, cartilage, skin and tendons, and
elastin is mainly responsible for the elastic properties of the
blood vessels, lungs and skin.

Dr. Hendler also points out that copper is known to
help protect against the ravages of oxygen-induced damage
to body tissues, through an enzyme called copper-zinc

superoxide dismutase and a protein called ceruloplasmin. Both have known anti-inflammatory effects in the body. Further, copper seems to play an important role in maintaining the structural integrity of the cell membranes. "Copper's folk-remedy reputation as an anti-arthritic agent may turn out to have some scientific validity," Dr. Hendler says.

Rather than wearing a copper bracelet or taking huge amounts of this nutrient, "for now, the best thing you can do is to make sure you are within the estimated safe and adequate range of 1.5 to 3 mg. of copper a day in your diet, whether you have arthritis or not," says David Milne, Ph.D., a researcher in trace minerals at the U.S. Department of Agriculture Human Nutrition Research Center. No RDA has been established for this nutrient.

Q: You mean I might not be getting enough copper?

A: Studies show that only about 17 percent of people in the United States get 2 to 3 mg. a day of copper. In one study, women were getting about 1 mg. and men, 1.6 mg.

Q: What are good food sources of copper?

A: Liver, oysters, crabmeat, shiitake mushrooms, sesame and sunflower seeds, and nuts all contain good amounts of copper. Remember, though, as with other trace minerals, large doses of copper are toxic. You should take copper supplements only with medical supervision.

Q: You said earlier that taking NSAIDs can increase a person's need for vitamin C. Do any other arthritis drugs deplete your body of particular nutrients?

A: Methotrexate, a drug used for RA, actually works by depleting the body of a B-complex vitamin, folic acid. Some studies show that adding folic acid reduces methotrexate's side effects without affecting the drug's effectiveness.

People with RA taking nonsteroidal anti-inflammatory drugs have been found to have reduced blood levels of zinc.

Steroid drugs, too, such as prednisone, tend to deplete bone mass, especially if they are taken in large doses or over a long period of time. To attempt to counteract that, some doctors tell their patients on steroids to get extra amounts of calcium and vitamin D. Finally, penicillamine, gold and steroids may all interfere with the body's ability to absorb and use selenium and other trace minerals, including copper.

Q: So far you've talked only about rheumatoid arthritis. What are the dietary recommendations for people with osteoarthritis?

A: The top dietary recommendation for osteoarthritis is to maintain your normal weight. Several population studies have shown a link between obesity and the development of osteoarthritis, mostly in the weight-bearing joints, the hips and knees, and even the feet and ankles.

Q: What exactly is this link?

A: Those joints take a lot of abuse from added weight, explains Wilson Hayes, Ph.D., a professor of biomechanics at Harvard Medical School and director of the Orthopedic Biomechanics Laboratory at Beth Israel Hospital, in Boston. "If you stand on one leg, you generate about three times your body weight on your hip, knee and ankle;

if you climb or descend stairs, you are putting roughly six times your body weight on these joints. So for every extra pound, the force goes up proportionately," he says.

A knee joint can actually be compressed from extra weight, making the cartilage-lined bones grind against each other and causing excessive wear and tear. Heavy thighs can contribute to pain by forcing you to stand with your feet far apart and your toes pointed out. That stance throws your joints out of alignment and adds stress to hips and knees.

Q: Can losing weight prevent osteoarthritis?

A: A recent study indicates that, yes, it can. To find out if weight loss can prevent osteoarthritis, researchers at Boston University School of Medicine reviewed the weight histories of 64 women recently diagnosed with osteoarthritis of the knee and 728 women without the condition. (All the women had been weighed frequently as participants in the Framingham Study, an ongoing landmark study that has followed the health of the residents of Framingham, Massachusetts, for 44 years.) The study showed that an overweight woman of average height (5'3") who loses 11 pounds over a 10-year-period can reduce her risk of developing knee arthritis by more than half. And women who lose more weight decrease their arthritis risk even further.

"This study suggests that a large number of overweight women might delay or even prevent osteoarthritis of the knee if they lose weight," says Lawrence Shulman, M.D., director of the National Institute of Arthritis and Musculo-skeletal and Skin Diseases.

Q: But can losing weight help people who already have osteoarthritis?

A: There are no good studies to prove that losing weight lessens joint pain or slows the progress of the disease in people who already have osteoarthritis. But the experience of doctors who treat people with osteoarthritis is that weight loss does help, simply by taking the squeeze off over-burdened joints, says Robert P. Sheon, M.D., a senior rheuma-tologist and clinical professor of medicine at the Medical College of Ohio.

"To see this effect, though, you have to be at least 20 per-cent above ideal body weight to begin with, and you have to lose at least half your excess weight," Dr. Sheon says. "So someone who's 300 pounds has to lose at least 60 pounds before he or she is going to notice an appreciable benefit."

Q: I've heard that people who are severely overweight often don't do well with artificial joints. Is that true?

A: In general, they don't seem to do as well as people of normal weight, Dr. Sheon says.

Doctors have been reluctant to do joint replacements in people who are very big and heavy, because cemented joints are more likely to loosen in people who weigh more than 180 pounds.

With the new cementless joints, however, this may prove to be less of a problem, Dr. Sheon says. But there's no data yet to show the success rates at 5 or 10 years for these cementless joints in big people. "I feel strongly there should be restric-tions," Dr. Sheon says. "I see too many complications in people who weigh more than 180 pounds."

Q: What about people with rheumatoid arthritis? Does losing weight ever help them?

A: As we said earlier, people with RA tend to be about 10 pounds underweight. Studies show that those who are overweight, however, do seem to increase their risk for joint damage. Their inflamed joints simply can't handle the load. So it's probable that they, too, would benefit from weight loss.

Q: You talked so much about fish oils and rheumatoid arthritis? Do fish oils provide any benefit for people with osteoarthritis?

A: Osteoarthritis is much less likely than rheumatoid arthritis to be associated with inflammation, and that's why fish oils and evening-primrose oil aren't usually recommended for this condition. But in one small study, British researchers did try adding fish oil to some of their osteoarthritic patients' regular treatments with ibuprofen. At four months, the people taking the fish oil had "strikingly lower" assessment of pain and interference with daily activities than the patients taking ibuprofen alone, according to the report.

Q: What about the nutrients you mentioned earlier that help keep bones strong or that are important for cartilage formation? Can they do anything for osteoarthritis?

A: Here again, evidence is scant, and many of the studies that have been done over the years simply aren't up to the rigorous standards today's medical community demands as proof that something works. Rather than looking for one particular nutrient to cure your disease, your best bet is to make sure you really are getting the RDA of every nutrient. Many nutrients are important for bone health: calcium, vitamins D, C and B_6, pantothenic acid, boron, copper, fluoride, magnesium and others.

Of the few studies that have been done, two by British researchers showed an improvement in symptoms of osteoarthritis with supplemental pantothenic acid.

Vitamin C has proven helpful, in an animal study, in preventing cartilage damage. And vitamin C has been found to increase cartilage cell growth in rabbits.

Vitamin E was found helpful in relieving pain from osteoarthritis in a study by Israeli researchers. More than half of the 32 patients taking 600 I.U. of vitamin E a day for 10 days experienced marked relief of pain, according to this study.

Q: Aren't there nutritional supplements I can take to help my body rebuild cartilage?

A: There are substances being sold with the claim that they can rebuild cartilage, but again, sadly, the proof that they work is mostly overseas studies that most U.S. researchers would regard as not proof enough. Substances like green-lipped mussels, shark cartilage and calf cartilage, along with a substance called **chondroitin sulfate**, all contain building blocks for cartilage—**glycosaminoglycans**. Chondroitin sulfate is popular in Europe and Japan, and is available in some health-food stores. Studies in Europe and Japan have shown benefits in restoring damaged cartilage, both with oral and injected forms of chondroitin sulfate. Dr. Hendler calls chondroitin sulfate "a promising substance that deserves further research."

OTHER ALTERNATIVE TREATMENTS

Q: Isn't there some sort of liquid that people put on their joints to ease pain?

A: You're talking about DMSO, which is short for dimethyl sulfoxide. DMSO has been used since the 1940s as an industrial solvent, and was introduced into therapeutic practice in the 1960s. It was studied by researchers for a time for a variety of problems, ranging from athletic injuries to rheumatoid arthritis.

DMSO is odorless and colorless, but once applied to a joint, it can leave your breath smelling of garlic, onions or worse. Many claims have been made as to its proposed modes of action, but none of these claims have been widely accepted, Dr. Hendler says.

The Arthritis Survey found that DMSO provided temporary relief of joint pain in about half the 47 people who tried it. It is not recommended, though, since it does not outperform standard arthritis treatments, and it has not been proven to affect the course of the disease.

Dr. Hendler suggests that if you do use DMSO, you use only medical grade DMSO prescribed by a doctor. He says the DMSO sold in many stores and on the street should be avoided: It is almost never of the relatively pure grade used in clinical trials, and potential contaminants in street-grade DMSO pose a real risk.

After a review of the research studies done on DMSO, a special committee of the National Academy of Sciences found DMSO too "iffy" and too risky to become a prescription drug, much less an over-the-counter drug. In animals, DMSO has caused damage to the lens of the eye. In 1978, however, the Food and Drug Administration approved DMSO for one treatment—a bladder disease called interstitial cystitis (fibrosis of the bladder wall, occurring primarily in women over 40). And its use for a number of skin, nerve and auto-immune diseases is being investigated. But there are still no studies to prove that DMSO does anything to help arthritis.

Q: What about bee venom? I've heard some people with rheumatoid arthritis are treated with it.

A: Bee venom has a long history of use as a folk remedy for inflammatory conditions, such as rheumatoid arthritis. But there are no controlled clinical studies proving it works. There are some anecdotal reports and uncontrolled studies, however, that indicate benefits.

Dr. Panush, writing in *A Primer on the Rheumatic Diseases* (Atlanta: The Arthritis Foundation, 1988) has this to say about venom therapies: "Bee, ant and other venoms have been considered for treating patients with RA. Bee venoms are rich in phospholipase and other anti-inflammatory substances. They suppressed the development of experimental arthritis but have not been shown to affect the disease in humans. . . . Some venoms may eventually provide a novel and useful mode of antirheumatic therapy."

Twenty-three people in the Arthritis Survey tried bee stings for their arthritis, and 48 percent found it effective. That same number found it ineffective. Four percent said it made them feel worse.

If you are interested in bee-venom therapy for treatment of rheumatoid arthritis or other inflammatory conditions, you may be able to find a medical doctor, an osteopath or a doctor of Oriental medicine who offers bee-venom therapy. The venom is injected just under your skin. You must have a series of injections over the course of months, in slowly increasing amounts, and after about six treatments you may receive as many as 20 to 30 injections per visit, says Christopher Kim, M.D., of the Monmouth Pain Center, in Red Bank, New Jersey.

However, according to him, if the treatment is going to work, you should start to feel results within three visits. Dr. Kim has conducted several uncontrolled studies with bee venom in the treatment of rheumatoid arthritis, osteoarthritis, fibromyositis (inflammation of fibromuscular tissue) and some types of neuritis, and is the author of a textbook on bee-venom therapy, written in both English and Korean for doctors of Oriental and Western medicine.

It's also possible to get the venom straight from the bees. That's a service Charles Mraz, of Vermont, has been providing for more than 50 years to people with arthritis. A beekeeper who got relief from his own arthritis years ago by being stung by honeybees, he says he's seen it work. "I couldn't tell you exactly how many people have come here for help," he says. "Thousands."

Q: **How long does it take for people to see results?**

A: "That depends on what type of arthritis they have and how bad they have it. All sorts of factors are involved," Mraz says. "Sometimes a few treatments clear it up, and sometimes it takes a long time." He says he must sometimes give as many as 2,000 to 3,000 stings over the course of a year or more to get good results. (For more information about bee-venom therapy, contact the American Apitherapy Society, P.O. Box 74, North Hartland, VT 05052; (802) 295-8764.

Q: What about acupuncture? A friend of mine gets acupuncture treatments once a week and says they have eased her osteoarthritis pain.

A: Acupuncture is a Chinese therapy that involves inserting very fine, sterilized needles into certain areas of the body. It's not considered painful, and the risks are minor—only a slight risk of infection if the needles are not properly sterilized. (Some doctors use disposable needles.)

Acupuncture does seem to have pain-relieving effects, although just how it works on pain isn't understood. Some researchers believe it stimulates the body's production of natural painkillers or anti-inflammatory biochemicals. The Chinese say it stimulates "vital energy" in the body—restoring energy imbalances, breaking up energy blockages and helping the body to heal itself.

Q: But is there any proof that acupuncture works?

A: A recent study by Danish researchers compared the pain-relieving abilities of acupuncture with standard drug therapy in a group of 29 people with severe knee osteoarthritis who were candidates for knee-replacement surgery. Half the patients were randomly assigned to receive acupuncture treatments; the other half received standard painkillers.

The researchers measured pain relief and knee function, including the time it took to walk 50 feet and climb 20 steps on a staircase. They also measured range of motion and muscle strength. After nine weeks, the people receiving acupuncture treatments had significantly less pain and better function than those on analgesics, according to the researchers. In fact, seven people responded so well they declined surgery.

These researchers followed 17 of the initial 29 patients, continuing to give them acupuncture once a month for a year. With some ups and down, these patients were able to maintain the improvements seen at the beginning of the treatment.

While this all sounds good, American researchers say these results need to be repeated in other studies before this treatment can be considered proven to work.

Q: Anything else on acupuncture?

A: The Arthritis Survey turned up some interesting findings. The results, as a whole, showed that acupuncture provided little more relief than would be expected from a placebo. Some 37 percent said the treatment eased their pain. But when the researchers looked at a subset of the people who had acupuncture—in particular, those who'd gotten their treatment from a bona fide acupuncturist, not a chiropractor or M.D. dabbling in the technique—the good results doubled, to 73 percent!

Q: How do I find someone who does acupuncture treatments?

A: If you're considering acupuncture, look for a practitioner who is either state-licensed or certified by the National Commission for the Certification of Acupuncturists, 1424 16th St. N.W., Suite 501, Washington, DC 20036; (202) 232-1404. For a directory of certified acupuncturists in your state, send your request in writing, along with $3. For a national directory, send $18.

The American Association of Acupuncture and Oriental Medicine can also provide a referral to a licensed acupuncturist in your area. Contact this group at 4101 Lake Boone Tr., Suite 201, Raleigh, NC 27607; (919) 787-5181.

Q: Do any herbal remedies help arthritis?

A: No doubt many have been tried, but here again, there are few controlled clinical trials to prove that any work. One remedy that has caught researchers' attention is a Chinese herb called ***Triptergium wilfordii***, or thundervine root. In a study by researchers at Peking Union Medical College Hospital, in Beijing, this herb showed encouraging activity in people with rheumatoid arthritis. An extract of the plant achieved a 90 percent reduction in pain and other RA symptoms in 30 patients who were treated for 12 weeks.

A control group that received harmless placebos showed only 23 percent improvement. The observable clinical benefits were accompanied by improvements in the biochemical factors associated with RA, including rheumatoid factor and some measures of immune function.

There were some side effects, however, from the thundervine extract—mainly skin rashes and mild diarrhea. Several of the women found that the drug stopped their menstrual periods. In a few postmenopausal women, the drug brought on bleeding.

Chinese researchers continue to look at this herb, hoping to isolate its helpful components. But don't look for thundervine at your local health-food store. By law, American herbalists are prohibited from prescribing it.

Q: Can herbs be dangerous?

A: They certainly can. Just like drugs, all herbs, essential oils and extracts can contain active ingredients that cause serious side effects if they are not used properly. And there's been at least one confirmed case where a remedy being marketed as ''Chinese herbs'' turned out to include more than just herbs. When analyzed, these little black balls were found to contain indomethacin, a strong anti-inflammatory drug with a long list of potential side effects, and prednisone, a steroid drug with its own possible side effects.

EXPERIMENTAL TREATMENTS

Q: What's considered an experimental treatment? And how is it different from an alternative treatment such as acupuncture?

A: Most researchers consider an experimental treatment one that is being actively investigated in controlled clinical trials. A controlled trial is a study in which one group of people get the treatment being studied, while a similar group, the control group, gets either a placebo treatment or the standard treatment. Researchers consider an alternative treatment one that is not being investigated in any official, organized manner.

But even the medical profession has trouble discerning the difference.

"Sometimes there may be a fine line between an experimental and an alternative treatment, and a treatment that for a long time has been considered alternative, such as fish oils, may move into the experimental category and eventually become an accepted treatment," says John Klippel, M.D., clinical director of the National Institute of Arthritis and Musculoskeletal and Skin Diseases.

Q: What kinds of experimental treatments are being investigated now for arthritis?

A: There are many different areas of study. They include the development of what are called **biologicals**, medicinal preparations derived from living organisms, which are administered in the same manner as drugs and alter the body's immune response; new drugs that fight inflammation, hopefully with fewer side effects than the drugs being used currently; drugs already approved for use that may also be effective against arthritis; and even biochemical agents that may stimulate cartilage regrowth.

Arthritis research has benefitted tremendously from basic research being done in the areas of cancer, organ transplantation and AIDS, adds Dr. Klippel. "Both cancer drugs and the drugs used to prevent the rejection of organ transplants are being tried in people with rheumatoid arthritis."

Methotrexate, for instance, was first used as a cancer drug before it was tried, in much smaller doses, as a treatment for rheumatoid arthritis. And **cyclosporine**, a drug used to prevent rejection in organ-transplant patients, has been used with some success in people with rheumatoid arthritis who haven't responded well to other treatments.

Dr. Klippel also believes that the antiviral drugs used in the treatment of AIDS may one day provide benefits to people with rheumatoid arthritis. "Many people suspect that a virus may be the initiating factor in RA, and so an antiviral drug may help the body fight the disease process," he says.

Q: Sounds like there are many research studies going on? Are there?

A: Nobody knows exactly how many studies of experimental treatments for arthritis are being conducted at any one time, but it's in the dozens, not hundreds. That's because drug companies and biotechnology companies—those producing the biologicals—tend to be secretive about what they're studying. They don't want their competitors stealing their good ideas. Right now, NIAMS is funding only one major clinical trial, on a form of tetracycline called **minocycline**, which we'll describe in a minute. NIAMS is also currently funding several small pilot studies "and lots of basic background research," Dr. Klippel says.

Q: How does someone become involved in a research study?

A: The best way to find out about research studies, both private and federally funded, is to ask your doctor to contact the nearest NIAMS-sponsored multidisciplinary arthritis center (see page 170), Dr. Klippel says. Researchers at an arthritis center can tell your doctor if the center is currently enrolling participants for a study. If it is and if it sounds like you might qualify, the researchers will review your medical records. After that, if it still looks like you might qualify, you will then go to the center for an examination and to discuss the study.

Most of the people who enroll in arthritis-research studies are required to live within an hour's drive of the research facility, says Dr. Grayzel of the Arthritis Foundation. That's because the studies are done on an outpatient basis, and the researchers want to make sure the participants show up every two weeks or so.

You can also send for a free copy of the publication *New Medicines in Development for Arthritis* by the Pharmaceutical Manufacturers Association, 1100 15th St. N.W., Washington, DC 20005. This newsletter lists drugs that are currently under FDA review or are in human clinical trials for rheumatoid arthritis, osteoarthritis, gout, juvenile rheumatoid arthritis, lupus, osteoporosis, scleroderma and spondylitis. It lists the company making the drug but does not indicate where research is being done.

Q: How can I evaluate an experimental treatment?

A: By law, the researchers are required to discuss in detail the possible risks involved in any research study, and their study in particular, with anyone considering enrolling in the study.

Because it is an experimental treatment, there may not be much published about it. Still, you'll want to know what has been published, including animal studies and studies by foreign researchers. Find out: How long has this treatment been studied? How many studies have been done? Where? Any at prestigious universities? How many people have used this treatment to date? Will I be the first? The hundredth? What are the studies showing in terms of benefits? What kinds of side effects are appearing? Have any deaths been associated with this treatment? Are there a lot of things the researchers just don't know about this treatment?

Remember, new is not necessarily better. Although some promising treatments seem to be in the works, experience has proved that there are always a few dogs as well. As one researcher puts it, "A lot of treatments look promising at the start, but many are found to have problems that limit their use." The clinical trials are designed to uncover at least some of the problems.

Many researchers think biologicals hold the most hope for specific and effective therapies for rheumatoid arthritis, perhaps even a cure. So let's look at them first.

Q: What exactly is a biological?

A: As we said earlier, a biological is a medicinal preparation (researchers call them agents, not drugs) made from living organisms and their products. Most are derived from mouse or human immune cells.

All the biologicals being studied for arthritis have some sort of effect on the body's immune system: either to restore normal function, to alter function or to suppress a function.

Q: **What are biologicals supposed to do in the case of RA?**

A: Unfortunately, no one knows for sure what biologicals need to do in order to be effective against RA and other rheumatic diseases, so researchers are trying all sorts of biologicals with all sorts of immune-system actions. Most biologicals, however, have some sort of effect on T-cells, immune cells thought to play an important role in the inflammatory process of RA.

One reason for the confusion is that no one knows exactly how the immune-system functions in the case of RA, so no one knows for sure what immune-system functions need to be altered to have an impact on this disease, explains Nathan Zvafler, M.D., professor of medicine at the University of California at San Diego. "If basic investigators could tell the biotechnology industry what to make to cure one or another rheumatic disease, I am sure a biological that does cure the disease could be developed within a six-month period," Dr. Zvafler says.

Q: **What sorts of biologicals are being tried right now?**

A: One that's gone through at least eight clinical trials with RA patients is **gamma-interferon**, a biological that's used in another form (alpha) as a treatment for some types of cancer.

Gamma-interferon is a protein produced by certain of the body's immune cells when they are invaded by viruses. Interferon itself is not an antiviral agent, but it acts to stimulate noninfected cells, causing them to make another protein with antiviral characteristics. Interferon can also be produced by cells in response to a wide variety of stimulants, including bacteria. Interferon also has other effects on the body's immune system. Its role in rheumatoid arthritis is unclear.

In studies in which gamma-interferon has been given to people with rheumatoid arthritis, results have been mixed. In these studies, improvement in symptoms of joint swelling and pain ranged from 15 to 60 percent, says Grant Cannon, M.D., assistant professor of medicine at the University of Utah, in Salt Lake City. Dr. Cannon has done some of that research himself.

Q: Any other new research?

A: Another area of research is in **monoclonal antibodies**. An antibody, you'll recall, is a type of blood protein made by the body in response to a foreign substance (called an antigen). An antibody binds to an antigen and eliminates it from the body. Monoclonal antibodies are all exactly the same, reproduced by the zillions in a laboratory. (They are grown from tumor cells.)

Arthritis researchers are interested in certain types of monoclonal antibodies because they seem to be capable of blocking inflammatory reactions by certain cells, including cells in the joint capsule. Unlike most anti-inflammatory drugs used for arthritis, monoclonal antibodies seem to provide their beneficial effects right at the source of the action—certain immune cells that get into a joint and produce inflammation.

Just how well monoclonal-antibody therapy may work for RA has yet to be determined. Studies done so far, with a variety of antibodies, have been mostly favorable, says Arthur Kavanaugh, M.D., a rheumatologist at the University of Texas Southwestern Medical School, in Dallas.

A study done by researchers at that school used a monoclonal antibody called anti-CD-54 (Yes, they all have letters and numbers—pretty confusing!) The antibody was given to 13 people with severe, long-standing rheumatoid arthritis. Nine participants noted marked improvement as early as the eighth day of treatment. Six participants sustained improvement for a period of greater than two months. Side effects were minimal. They included nausea, fever and headaches, which resolved despite continued therapy.

"Treatment for RA has always been very capricious—kind of a shotgun approach," Dr. Kavanaugh explains. "With therapies such as this, hopefully we may be better able to design treatments aimed at the actual pathology, or cause, of the disease."

Q: What other kinds of biologicals are being tried?

A: There are several, but one type in particular—**immunotoxins**—have gotten people's interest. Immunotoxins start out as monoclonal antibodies but are combined with a toxin so that when they attach to a cell's surface they destroy the cell. So far, immunotoxins have been designed to destroy T-cells, which, as we said earlier, are immune cells thought to play a major role in inflammation. It may be possible, however, to design an immunotoxin that can destroy any type of cell.

In one study by researchers at the University of California at San Francisco, 18 of 20 RA patients had 50 percent or greater improvement in joint pain following a single treatment with an immunotoxin developed by the Xoma Corporation, in Berkeley. In a Harvard University study, 12 of 13 people with severe rheumatoid arthritis that hadn't responded to other therapies showed a significant response to an immunotoxin containing deactivated diphtheria toxin.

Studies of immunotoxins are ongoing, but researchers say it's too soon to know if these agents can provide long-term relief.

Q: What about anti-inflammatory drugs? Are there any safer, more effective ones being developed?

A: We don't know about safer or more effective, but there certainly are a lot of anti-inflammatory drugs being marketed, and manufacturers keep coming out with more of them.

At least a dozen new anti-inflammatory drugs are currently being tested or are awaiting FDA approval to be marketed, according to the Pharmaceutical Manufacturers Association. To be given approval, a drug must prove that it is at least as safe and effective as those in the same category already on the market. So clinical trials must compare the drug with others in its class. Even though an FDA-approved drug may have appeared to be safe and effective in clinical trials, usually not until it's been on the market for a few years and been used by tens of thousands of people do its real strengths and weaknesses reveal themselves. That's one reason some doctors like to avoid prescribing new drugs to their patients.

One anti-inflammatory drug, tenidap sodium, was mentioned in the *NIAMS 1992 Research Highlights*, an annual journal. This drug seems to be unique among NSAIDs in that it has a dual anti-inflammatory action. In addition to inhibiting the body's manufacture of inflammatory prostaglandins, the drug acts on immune cells called neutrophils, which, when activated, release biochemicals that can damage cells, say researchers at the University of Alabama. Neutrophils are the predominant cells in synovial fluid, and are frequently found in areas where inflamed, proliferating synovial tissue is pressing against cartilage.

This drug has more than held its own against three other popular NSAIDs, and is currently being tested in a large trial of 10,000 people. Further study should show whether or not this drug helps to alter the progressive joint damage so commonly seen in patients with arthritis. Tenidap sodium is currently being considered for use in either osteoarthritis or rheumatoid arthritis, its manufacturer says.

Q: You said earlier that tetracycline was being tried in people with rheumatoid arthritis. What's the story behind that?

A: Researchers at NIAMS are now testing a form of the antibiotic tetracycline, called minocycline, on 219 people with rheumatoid arthritis.

An Israeli study tested minocycline in people with rheumatoid arthritis and found significant improvements in almost all aspects of the disease.

Antibiotics have been tried, off and on, for the treatment of arthritis for about 30 years, but so far, studies of their effectiveness have been mixed, says Stephen Heyse, M.D., director of the office of prevention, epidemiology and clinical application at NIAMS.

"We are looking at this drug not for its antibiotic effect, but for other effects," Dr. Heyse says. "Certain antibiotics alter the immune system in a way that reduces inflammation. This particular drug, for instance, seems to inhibit an enzyme that is involved in dissolving cartilage in the joint."

Minocycline may prove to be useful for the treatment of RA, but like other drugs, it does have side effects. Dizziness, nausea and rashes were most commonly reported by the Israeli researchers. "And we are concerned that its long-term use may enhance the growth of antibiotic-resistant micro-organisms in the body," Dr. Heyse says. In the Israeli study, three people developed either oral or skin yeast infections.

5 OTHER QUESTIONS ABOUT ARTHRITIS

Q: My friend claims her rheumatoid arthritis has gotten better since she started estrogen-replacement therapy. Is there any proof this should help?

A: One study, by researchers at the University of California at San Francisco, found that women with rheumatoid arthritis who take estrogen-replacement therapy have milder symptoms than women who took estrogen in the past but stopped or who never used estrogen.

The study of 154 postmenopausal women with RA found that use of estrogen-replacement therapy was associated with significantly fewer painful joints and better performance of daily activities.

Sex hormones are steroids, which are known to influence immune response and the course of autoimmune diseases. (Such diseases are more common in women of reproductive age.) Just what role sex hormones may play in rheumatoid arthritis remains to be determined, researchers say. Pregnancy improves RA symptoms for women. And some evidence suggests that the use of oral contraceptives can reduce a woman's lifetime risk for RA, or at least delay its onset.

Q: But aren't there risks associated with estrogen replacement therapy?

A: There are risks, so you'll need to be carefully monitored by your doctor if you decide to take estrogen and other replacement hormones.

Estrogen, when taken alone in any form, increases a woman's risk of developing cancer of the endometrium—

the uterine lining. So a woman should take an additional hormone, progesterone, which causes the uterine lining to be shed each month. If she does not take progesterone, her doctor should occasionally take a sample of endometrium to make sure it is normal.

Studies that look at the risk for breast cancer in women taking estrogen replacement hormones have been mixed. Most have found no increased risk. One study, however, found a slightly increased risk of 10 percent overall and also found several high-risk groups. Women who took a combination of estrogen and progesterone for more than six years, for instance, appeared to have 4.4 times the average risk of developing breast cancer. That was a very small group, though, and doctors say additional research is needed to learn more about the risks of such long-term therapy. A doctor will probably recommend a yearly mammogram for any woman undergoing estrogen replacement therapy.

Q: Will moving to a warmer climate help my arthritis?

A: Studies on the effect of weather on rheumatoid arthritis show that when barometric pressure goes down and humidity goes up, the symptoms of arthritis worsen for some people. And many people say their joints feel better when the weather is warm and dry than when it's cold and damp.

The weather itself doesn't cause arthritis, however, and it's unlikely that moving to a warmer climate will alter the course of the disease, although it may make you feel more comfortable. Before you pick up and move, it's a good idea to visit a place for a few weeks to see if you really do feel better being there. Some people with arthritis who move to a new climate find that the disadvantages of giving up their ties to family and friends outweigh the advantages of a sunny clime.

Q: What exactly is rheumatism?

A: It's an imprecise term people used to describe just about any condition that causes pain and swelling in joints and surrounding tissues. Rheumatism may be diagnosed as arthritis, bursitis or any other number of painful conditions.

Q: Is there a connection between stress and arthritis?

A: There does seem to be a connection, researchers are discovering. "It's common to encounter people with rheumatoid arthritis who relate the onset of their symptoms with a particularly stressful period in their lives, or who say their symptoms flare up when they are feeling stressed," says Ronald Wilder, M.D., chief of the inflammatory-joint-disease section at the National Institute of Arthritis and Musculo-skeletal and Skin Diseases.

Q: How might stress play a role in arthritis?

A: One theory is that people who develop chronic inflammation may have a stress-hormone deficiency, says Esther Sternberg, M.D, chief of the neuroendocrine, immunology and behavior unit at the National Institute of Mental Health. "They appear to produce lower levels of corticosteroids, which are normally released by the adrenal glands in response to physical or emotional stress, and which are the most potent anti-inflammatory agents produced by the body," she says.

In animal studies, the inability to produce normal amounts of corticosteroids has been associated with the development of inflammatory diseases after exposure to inflammation-producing agents, Dr. Sternberg says. Animals who can produce a burst of these hormones during exposure to inflammation-producing agents tend not to develop chronic inflammation.

Q: So why would someone have a stress-hormone deficiency?

A: That's the million-dollar question, Dr. Sternberg says. "We know that in some rats it's a genetic problem, but we also know we can take normal rats and hinder their ability to produce corticosteroids by giving them certain drugs or by removing their adrenal glands. In humans, it's probably a variety of factors that produce this problem."

Q: How can I find out if I have this deficiency myself?

A: It is possible to have a test that measures your blood levels of stress hormones, but currently your doctor is likely to have trouble using the test results to predict the course of your RA or to offer treatment, according to Dr. Sternberg. Testing standards that would associate certain blood levels of stress hormones with symptoms of inflammation have yet to be developed.

Q: So what can I do if I think stress is contributing to my symptoms?

A: Researchers say this:

• Don't be embarrassed if your condition varies with the amount of stress you feel. It may have a very real basis.

• Avoid what stressful situations you can. "Stress management, psychological counseling or biofeedback may help you react less to stressful situations, but they are not going to change what may be an underlying physiological problem," Dr. Sternberg says.

• Based on the theory that many people with RA may have a stress-hormone deficiency, some doctors prescribe what they call physiological doses (3 to 4 milligrams a day) of steroid drugs. They allow their patients to assess their own degree of inflammation and determine their own dosage. That's something Dr. Wilder does, and the one study done so far on this use of steroids seems to show it works fairly well at relieving symptoms, with few side effects.

• Some doctors also prescribe antidepressants, which seem to help normalize either overproduction or underproduction of corticosteroids.

Q: I know that smoking cigarettes increases my risks of developing heart disease and cancer. Does smoking also increase my chances of developing arthritis?

A: A study by researchers in Finland suggests that smoking can dramatically up your odds for developing rheumatoid arthritis, but only if you're a man. The study found that male smokers are almost eight times more likely to develop rheumatoid arthritis than nonsmokers. Even ex-smokers have a higher risk—they are four times more prone to RA than men who have never smoked. The Finnish study is drawn from data on more than 57,000 people who've been followed since 1966. In that time, over 500 have developed RA; of the male arthritis sufferers, only five had never smoked.

The researchers speculate that exposure to smoke triggers the release of rheumatoid factor, which combines with male hormones to contribute to the development of the disease.

Q: Does depression have something to do with RA?

A: Researchers say it's common for people with rheumatoid arthritis to have what's called *atypical depression*, a form characterized by foul moods, lack of energy and excessive sleep.

"This has been noted for many years, but it tended to be seen as secondary to the arthritis—simply as a normal reaction to having a serious disease," Dr. Sternberg says.

However, research by the National Institute of Mental Health suggests that this depression may be caused by the same stress-hormone deficiency that increases people's susceptibility to inflammatory illnesses. "It may be that people who have a tendency to develop rheumatoid arthritis have a similar tendency to develop certain kinds of depression under stress," Dr. Sternberg says.

Doctors are currently studying which types of antidepressants are most likely to help people with atypical depression. "We don't yet know which may help most, but it may be those that increase, rather than decrease, corticosteroid production," Dr. Sternberg says.

Q: **Can I have osteoarthritis and rheumatoid arthritis at the same time?**

A: Yes. Joints damaged by rheumatoid arthritis are prone to develop osteoarthritis, as are any injured joints. And RA-damaged weight-bearing joints, such as knees, are likely to develop osteoarthritis at an earlier-than-normal age. Both conditions need to be treated, using combinations of drugs that minimize RA flare-ups and relieve osteoarthritis pain, along with rest and non-weight-bearing exercises.

Q: **You mentioned Lyme disease earlier. Tell me again—what exactly is it? What causes it?**

A: Lyme disease is an infectious condition that can cause a number of medical problems, including arthritis, usually only in a few large joints.

It's caused by a spiral-shaped bacteria, called *Borrelia burgdorferi*, which is transmitted to humans by the bite of a deer tick, a tiny insect that in its immature state can fit on the head of a pin. Most people are bitten by immature ticks during spring and summer. Adult deer ticks are a little bigger and can bite at other times of the year.

Q: What are the symptoms of Lyme disease?

A: Its early symptoms can include a flulike illness, with chills, fever, headache, swollen glands and joint pain. About half of infected people also develop a distinctive rash around the site of the tick bite within three days to a month after being bitten. The rash often looks like a red ring with a clear center. The outer edges expand slowly in size. Sometimes the center of the ring becomes a large red blister.

If it is not treated, Lyme disease can cause severe nerve or heart problems, as well as arthritis.

Q: How is Lyme disease diagnosed?

A: Hopefully, your medical history can provide your doctor with enough clues for her to be fairly certain of a diagnosis. However, if you don't recall being bitten by a tick and do not develop the classic bull's-eye rash, diagnosis may be something of a challenge.

A number of blood tests can be done to test for Lyme disease. Most common are the indirect fluorescent antibody (IFA) test, the Western blot assay and the ELISA (enzyme-linked immunosorbent assay). All three measure antibodies in the blood formed against the bacteria that cause Lyme disease.

However, studies have shown that all three of these tests are inaccurate in detecting Lyme disease 20 to 60 percent of the time. Their false-positive or false-negative rates vary widely, depending in part on the laboratory at which they are done. That means you can't rely on a negative blood test to rule out the possibility that you have Lyme disease.

"Mounting evidence suggests that a significant number of people for some reason or another don't produce detectable antibodies in response to infection and thus are missed by the laboratory confirming tests that are available," says David Dorward, M.D., a senior staff fellow at the National Institute of Allergy and Infectious Diseases.

Just how many people with Lyme disease have negative blood tests is a matter of debate, says Kenneth Liegner, M.D., an internist from Armonk, New York, an area where Lyme disease is endemic. "Some doctors think it's quite rare, others think it's not rare at all," Dr. Liegner says. "I usually 'shotgun' it. I do several different tests, at several different labs, and see what I come up with. I put that together with the clinical picture to figure out what to do."

Q: Sounds like Lyme disease is often misdiagnosed. Is it?

A: It seems to be. "I think there are still a lot of people with Lyme disease falling through the cracks, while others who don't have Lyme are being told they do have it," Dr. Liegner says. If you think you may have this disease, he suggests you go to a Lyme Center associated with a teaching hospital. "Until recently, these centers tended to treat based only on blood tests, but that is changing now that evidence shows people may not develop detectable amounts of antibodies," Dr. Liegner says.

Some experts believe that a fair number of people seeking treatment for and being diagnosed as having Lyme disease actually have an arthritis-like condition called fibromyalgia. (In fact, though, other researchers have found fibromyalgia symptoms in people with confirmed Lyme disease.)

Q: How is Lyme disease treated?

A: In the early stages of the disease, oral antibiotics, such as doxycycline, amoxicillin and erythromycin, given for three to four weeks, are usually effective at curing Lyme disease. Intravenous antibiotics are often necessary in its later stages, and some people develop chronic symptoms that some doctors treat with long-term intravenous antibiotics.

Doctors who are familiar with the illness usually base their treatment decisions more on a person's symptoms than on blood tests, Dr. Liegner says. And they are more likely to treat a person with possible Lyme disease if the person lives in a state where the disease is common.

Q: Where is Lyme disease most common?

A: Eighty percent of the 40,000 cases reported since 1982 come from 10 states: New York, New Jersey, Connecticut, Pennsylvania, Massachusetts, Maryland, Rhode Island, Minnesota, Wisconsin and California. Scattered cases have been reported in just about every state.

Q: What can I do to protect myself from being bitten?

A: Experts suggest that when outdoors you should wear tightly woven light-colored clothing and tuck long pants into socks. Use a deet-containing insect repellent, using only enough to lightly spray your clothing and skin, especially your shoes, socks and lower pants legs.

When you come indoors, or once each day if you're outside for days at a time, check your body, including your groin and underarms, for ticks. Ask someone to check your head and neck. Check your pets daily for ticks. If you do find a tick, grasp it with fine-point tweezers as close to the skin as possible and pull it straight out. Do not attempt to crush it with your fingers. You can drive the hard shell into your skin. If possible, save the tick in a container filled with alcohol. That way, if you get sick, a doctor can identify the tick and more readily treat your illness.

If you know for sure you were bitten by a deer tick and you live in a high-risk state, some doctors suggest a preventive course of antibiotics even if you haven't developed symptoms.

Q: You said fibromyalgia is sometimes mistaken for Lyme disease. What's fibromyalgia?

A: This disorder literally means pain ("algia") in fibrous tissues, such as muscles, tendons and ligaments. It's also sometimes called fibrositis, but that name is misleading, since this condition does not involve inflammation. Some of its symptoms—chronic, diffuse aches and pains, disturbed sleep, morning fatigue and stiffness, headaches, numbness and/or tingling—are similar to those of arthritis, but standard arthritis treatments, such as nonsteroidal anti-inflammatory drugs, don't seem to help it.

Some 70 to 90 percent of people who develop fibromyalgia are women ages 20 to 50.

Q: How is fibromyalgia diagnosed?

A: The diagnosis is made on the basis of physical symptoms and the elimination of other possible disorders, such as Lyme disease and rheumatoid arthritis.

People with fibromyalgia have what doctors call "tender points" at specific locations throughout their bodies. These muscular nodules may not hurt spontaneously, but pressing on them causes pain. Doctors look for multiple tender points, which are uncommon in healthy people and in people with other rheumatic diseases.

There is no blood test or laboratory test to identify the presence of fibromyalgia. X-rays reveal nothing.

Q: Do doctors know what causes it?

A: No, but there are several theories. Some researchers think neurochemical abnormalities lead to sleep disturbances, which in turn lead to fatigue, pain and depression. Some think it's a problem of muscle energy metabolism, and that muscle cells starved for oxygen are causing the pain.

Others think it is caused by various infections, thyroid disease, head trauma or emotional stress. In fact, a recent study conducted at Tufts University School of Medicine, in Boston, concluded that some people have fibromyalgia triggered by Lyme disease. Of 287 people treated at a Lyme-disease clinic during a three-year period, 22 had fibromyalgia associated with Lyme disease. In another study, half of the people with fibromyalgia said their symptoms began after a flulike illness. Many had been misdiagnosed as having chronic-fatigue syndrome.

To confuse matters even more, some researchers think fibromyalgia and chronic-fatigue syndrome are the same condition.

Q: How is fibromyalgia treated?

A: Generally, nondrug treatments, such as heat, massage and muscle stretching, are tried first. Such treatments may be all some people require to relieve their symptoms. In one study, aerobic exercise was also helpful at relieving pain and improving sleep.

Antidepressants are the drugs used most often to treat fibromyalgia. This does not mean that people with fibromyalgia are depressed or have a psychiatric disorder. They are usually not depressed. Doctors prescribe these drugs, to be taken at bedtime, because they improve sleep and so eliminate some of the problems that poor sleep patterns can cause. In several studies, people taking either of two antidepressants, amitriptyline and cyclobenzaprine, showed a significant improvement in symptoms.

Doctors say that narcotics and steroid drugs should never be given to people with fibromyalgia.

Q: You've mentioned lupus a few times. What can you tell me about this disease?

A: Like rheumatoid arthritis, lupus is a chronic inflammatory disease in which the body's immune system forms antibodies that attack healthy tissues and organs. There are several types of lupus. **Discoid lupus** affects the skin, causing a butterfly-shaped rash across the face and a rash on the upper parts of the body. Systemic lupus erythematosus (SLE), usually more severe than discoid, can attack any body part, such as joints, kidneys, brain, heart and lungs. Like rheumatoid arthritis, lupus includes flare-ups and remissions. If not controlled, SLE can be fatal, but at least 90 percent of people with SLE live for at least 10 years after developing the disease.

Another form of this disease is drug-induced lupus, caused by reactions to medication. When the drug is stopped, the symptoms of lupus usually disappear.

It's not known how many people have discoid lupus. Probably many people have mild cases and don't know it. Researchers say there may be as many as 500,000 people with SLE in the United States, most of whom have not been correctly diagnosed.

Q: What causes lupus?

A: Only in the case of drug-induced lupus is the cause known. The drug most likely to be implicated is procainamide (Pronestyl), which is often used to treat heart irregularities. Other drugs known to cause lupus include hydralazine (a blood-pressure drug), isoniazid (used to treat tuberculosis), methyldopa (a blood-pressure drug), quinidine (used to treat heart irregularities) and chlorpromazine (used to treat psychosis and severe vomiting). There's also a long list of drugs that may possibly cause lupus, but researchers lack definite proof of the association.

It's thought that about 10 percent of people with lupus have drug-induced symptoms.

There seems to be a genetic tendency to develop lupus. In families of people with lupus, there is an increased incidence of both lupus and rheumatoid arthritis. That genetic tendency, along with exposure to certain viruses, chemicals in the environment or extreme emotional stress may trigger the immune process that leads to the formation of antibodies against the self.

Q: Who gets lupus?

A: Ninety percent of lupus patients are female. The disease affects one in 700 white females, and one in 250 black females.

Q: How is it diagnosed?

A: The skin rash of discoid lupus may be so typical that its appearance, along with a medical history, is enough to make a diagnosis. Someone with discoid lupus needs to have a complete physical examination, including laboratory tests to check for the possibility of SLE.

Diagnosing SLE is more difficult. A doctor who suspects lupus usually orders several blood tests that can detect various abnormal antibodies. The **antinuclear antibody (ANA) test** is a very useful screening test, because it is positive in at least 99 percent of people with systemic lupus. However, antinuclear antibodies may also be formed in reaction to certain medications, viral infections, liver diseases and various types of arthritis. So a positive result does not necessarily confirm that you have lupus, but a negative ANA test makes this diagnosis quite unlikely.

The blood test most commonly used to confirm the diagnosis of lupus detects antibodies to a person's own genetic material, DNA. This antibody can be found in the blood of about 75 percent of people with SLE, but it is rarely present in any other condition.

Q: How is lupus treated?

A: Discoid lupus may be treated with topical steroid creams and sunscreens. With more extensive skin disease, Plaquenil, the same antimalaria drug used to treat rheumatoid arthritis, is sometimes used, and seems to work quite well.

SLE has frequently been treated with long-term high-dose steroid drugs. But the vast majority of experts now say that most patients on high-dose steroids are paying too dearly for relief. Kidney failure and heart disease, the two conditions most likely to lead to death in people in lupus, have both been linked with the long-term use of steroid drugs. So experts recommend that steroids not be used unless major organs are immediately threatened with inflammation and destruction during disease flare-ups, and then only at the lowest effective dose. Less powerful drugs, including aspirin, nonsteroidal anti-inflammatory drugs and antimalaria drugs, can often control symptoms well enough. Or, in some cases, drugs that suppress the immune system may be used.

Q: What is juvenile rheumatoid arthritis?

A: Juvenile rheumatoid arthritis (JRA) is arbitrarily considered to be any kind of arthritis that begins before age 16. Juvenile rheumatoid arthritis is rare before the age of 6 months, and two onset peaks are generally observed, between the ages of 1 and 3 years and between 8 and 12 years. Girls are twice as likely as boys to develop JRA. There may be as many as 200,000 cases of juvenile rheumatoid arthritis in the United States, but no one knows its exact prevalence. In Britain, the prevalence is 1 in every 1,500 schoolchildren.

The symptoms of juvenile rheumatoid arthritis vary, and the disease is usually divided into three types: pauciarticular, polyarticular and systemic.

Q: What's the difference?

A: Pauciarticular arthritis means arthritis in only a few joints. This is the most common type of JRA, accounting for 40 to 50 percent of cases. In children age 5 or older, mild joint pain and swelling are often the only symptoms. Children age 5 or younger may also be listless and irritable, have a low-grade fever and fail to grow at a normal rate. One potentially serious manifestation of this type of arthritis is an inflammation of the iris of the eye, called iridocyclitis, which occurs in 20 to 30 percent of children. Children with this disorder need to have their eyes checked at least every three months by an ophthalmologist.

Polyarticular juvenile arthritis accounts for 30 to 40 percent of all cases of JRA. It is characterized by arthritis in more than four joints and can begin either abruptly or slowly. In either case, the child appears listless. He may refuse to eat and, subsequently, lose weight. Large joints, such as knees, wrists, ankles and elbows, are the most frequent sites of initial inflammation. The child may also have a low-grade fever, which may peak twice a day at no more than 102°.

Systemic juvenile rheumatoid arthritis, the least common type and the one type more likely to affect boys than girls, accounts for about 20 percent of cases of JRA. Its initial symptoms can vary. Sometimes there is simply joint pain, fever and a fleeting rash. In other cases there may be high fever, a rash, enlarged lymph glands and spleen, and often heart and lung inflammation.

Q: **What happens to children who develop juvenile rheumatoid arthritis?**

A: The overall prognosis for children with JRA is better than previously assumed. At least 75 percent eventually have long remissions without significant residual damage and presumably lead normal adult lives. Children with rheumatoid-factor positive or systemic-onset JRA are at greatest risk for chronic and destructive joint damage. Growth retardation occurs most frequently in children with chronic systemic arthritis or polyarticular arthritis.

Q: **Is juvenile rheumatoid arthritis treated the same way as adult RA?**

A: Not always. Nonsteroidal anti-inflammatory drugs, especially ibuprofen or aspirin, are the mainstays of treatment. Gold therapy may be started in children who haven't responded to NSAIDs within six months. Studies show that the toxicity in children is similar to that in adults and is of no greater severity or frequency. Hydroxychloroquine (Plaquenil) is sometimes used as an alternative to gold. Steroids drugs are avoided except in the case of life-threatening inflammation. Other drugs, such as methotrexate, have not been adequately studied in children. Many doctors think these drugs are too risky to use, since most children with JRA eventually go into remission with little permanent joint damage.

Q: What is scleroderma?

A: Scleroderma is a relatively rare form of arthritis that affects 50,000 to 100,000 people in the United States. It affects women three to four times more often than men, and its incidence increases steadily with age, most commonly with onset between ages 30 and 60.

Its name comes from the Greek word *sklero*, meaning hard, and derma, meaning skin. Many people with the disease develop areas of thick, rigid skin on their faces, fingers and arms. This disease is also called *progressive systemic sclerosis*, because it sometimes involves progressive hardening of tissue in other areas of the body, including joints, lungs, heart, kidneys and intestinal tract.

Scleroderma is a **collagen vascular disease**. Collagen is the fibrous tissue that gives resilience to skin and bones and that supports and connects other tissues in the body. In scleroderma, the body makes too much collagen, and the excess is deposited in the skin and other organs, resulting in hardness and tightness of the skin and possible organ dysfunction. The disease can also cause the abnormal growth of cells lining the blood vessels, which can cause vascular problems, such as the extreme sensitivity of the fingers to cold, a condition called *Raynaud's phenomenon*. The cause of this abnormal collagen growth is unknown. Like lupus, scleroderma is associated with abnormal antibodies that cause the body to attack its own tissue.

Q: What are the symptoms of scleroderma?

A: In most people, the first symptom is either Raynaud's phenomenon, hand swelling and puffiness, or pain and swelling in the joints of the hands. Skin thickening usually follows and may spread to other areas of the body. If joints, tendons and muscles become involved, pain, weakness and nerve compression may result. The gastrointestinal tract is frequently involved, and may cause swallowing problems, stomach pain and bloating. Changes in the lungs occur in about 40 percent of people, but few are incapacitated by this. Heart and kidney problems can also occur, and can be serious.

Q: How is scleroderma diagnosed?

A: There is no single test for this disease. Your doctor may order blood tests to rule out some other forms of arthritis and to check for certain types of antibodies. She may do tests to check the function of your lungs, heart, kidneys and gastrointestinal tract.

Q: How is scleroderma treated?

A: No single drug or combination of drugs has been demonstrated to be effective in controlling scleroderma. The use of steroids is usually restricted to severe inflammation. Immunosuppressive drugs have been tried, but reports of their effectiveness have been inconsistent. Nonsteroidal anti-inflammatory drugs are sometimes given to treat the arthritis symptoms associated with scleroderma. Other symptoms may be treated in a variety of ways. Drugs that dilate blood vessels may be used to improve circulation in tiny blood vessels and to help prevent high blood pressure and kidney damage. Heartburn may be treated with antacids, and problems with digesting and absorbing foods may mean you'll need to drink special nutrient-packed drinks.

Like rheumatoid arthritis, the course of scleroderma varies considerably. Overall, the 10-year-survival rate after first diagnosis is approximately 65 percent. The prognosis for this disease continues to improve, however, with the use of effective blood-pressure drugs that reduce the incidence of kidney failure.

Q: Haven't silicone breast implants been associated with scleroderma?

A: Silicone breast implants may be associated with some connective-tissue diseases, but one study reported no increased numbers of women with breast implants in a group of women with scleroderma. Most of the evidence that would connect silicone breast implants with scleroderma consists of anecdotal reports and reports of improvement in symptoms after breast implants are removed.

The most common symptoms associated with silicone breast implants seem to be fatigue and muscle and joint pain. An increased incidence of systemic sclerosis has been found in stonemasons and coal miners, who inhale silica dust.

INFORMATIONAL AND MUTUAL AID GROUPS

American Academy of Allergy and Immunology
611 E. Wells St.
Milwaukee, WI 53202
(414) 272-6071

Can refer you to a doctor in your area who diagnoses food allergies.

American Academy of Environmental Medicine
P.O. Box 16105
Denver, CO 80216
(303) 622-9755

Can refer you to a doctor in your area who diagnoses food allergies.

American Apitherapy Society
P.O. Box 74
North Hartland, VT 05052
(802) 295-8764

A nonprofit educational organization that provides information on bee venom therapy and bee products. No referrals to practitioners given.

American Association of Acupuncture and Oriental Medicine
4101 Lake Boone Tr.
Suite 201
Raleigh, NC 27607
(919) 787-5181

Provides referrals. Fee charged. For a directory of certified acupuncturists in up to three states, send request in writing, along with $5. Information packet also includes a patient brochure describing acupuncture and a list of other publications.

American College of Rheumatology
60 Executive Park S.
Suite 150
Atlanta, GA 30329
(404) 633-3777

Can tell you if a doctor is board-certified in rheumatology.

American Dietetic Association
430 N. Michigan Ave.
Chicago, IL 60611

For a list of registered dietitians in your area, send request in writing, along with a self-addressed stamped envelope and $1.

American Holistic Medical Association
2002 Eastlake Ave. E.
Seattle, WA 98102
(206) 322-6842

Can refer you to a doctor in your area who is a member of this organization.

American Nutritionists Association
P.O. Box 34030
Bethesda, MD 20817

For a list of nutrition consultants in your area, all of whom have advanced degrees in nutrition from reputable schools, send request in writing, along with a self-addressed stamped envelope and $1.

Ankylosing Spondylitis Association
511 N. LaCienega Blvd.
Suite 216
Los Angeles, CA 90048
(800) 777-8189
(310) 652-0609 (in California)

Provides information on this condition to consumers, health-care professionals and researchers. Maintains a library and conducts research.

Arthritis Foundation
1314 Spring St. N.W.
Atlanta, GA 30309
(800) 283-7800

Contact your local chapter, listed in the white pages of your phone book, to find out exactly what services are available in your area. Services may include information about arthritis; referrals to doctors and clinics; help in finding local services, such as home health care; classes on self-care; exercise classes; clubs or support groups for people with arthritis; discount drug services; and updates for health professionals on the latest research in improved care.

Food Allergy Network
4744 Holly Ave.
Fairfax, VA 22030-5647
(703) 691-3179

Send a self-addressed stamped envelope for a copy of the newsletter Food Allergy News *and a list of publications.*

Lupus Foundation of America
4 Research Pl.
Suite 180
Rockville, MD 20850-3226
(800) 558-0121

> *Provides information about lupus and can put callers in touch with support groups and treatment centers.*

National Chronic Pain Outreach Association
7979 Old Georgetown Rd.
Suite 100
Bethesda, MD 20814
(301) 652-4948

> *Provides information about chronic pain and its management. Operates an information clearinghouse for pain sufferers, family members and health-care professionals. A "Support Group Starter Kit" is available for the formation of local chronic-pain support groups.*

National Commission for the Certification of Acupuncturists
1424 16th St. N.W.
Suite 501
Washington, DC 20036
(202) 232-1404

> *Provides referrals. Fee charged. For a directory of certified acupuncturists in your state, send request in writing, along with $3. For a national directory, send $18.*

National Institute of Arthritis and Musculoskeletal and Skin Diseases
NIH Information Clearinghouse
Box AMS
9000 Rockville Pike
Bethesda, MD 20892
(301) 495-4484

> *Collects, publishes and disseminates professional and public educational materials for people concerned with arthritis and related conditions. Offers a computerized research service.*

NATIONAL INSTITUTE OF ARTHRITIS AND MUSCULOSKELETAL AND SKIN DISEASES MULTIPURPOSE CENTERS

The National Institute of Arthritis and Musculoskeletal and Skin Diseases (NIAMS) Multipurpose Centers develop and carry out programs in basic and/or clinical research as related to professional, patient and public education, epidemiology and health services. The centers are designed to develop new capabilities for research in these areas. The goal is to explore innovative new directions for understanding the causes, treatment and ultimate prevention of arthritis and musculoskeletal diseases.

The following centers, supported by NIAMS, are located throughout the country. Also listed are the center directors.

MIDDLE ATLANTIC

Cornell University Medical College
The Hospital for Special Surgery
Research Building, Room 605
535 East 70th St.
New York, NY 10021
(212) 606-1189
Director: Charles L. Christian, M.D.

MIDWEST

Case Western Reserve University
2074 Abington Rd.
Cleveland, OH 44106
(216) 844-3168
Director: Roland W. Moskowitz, M.D.

Indiana University School of Medicine
541 Clinical Dr., Room 492
Indianapolis, IN 46202-5103
(317) 274-4225
Director: Kenneth D. Brandt, M.D.

Northwestern University Medical School
303 E. Chicago Ave., Ward 3-315
Chicago, IL 60611
(313) 503-8197
Director: Richard M. Pope, M.D.

University of Michigan Medical Center
Taubman Health Care Center, Room 3918
Ann Arbor, MI 48109-0358
(313) 936-5566
Director: David A. Fox, M.D.

NEW ENGLAND

Brigham and Women's Hospital
75 Francis St.
Boston, MA 02115
(617) 732-5356
Director: Matthew H. Liang, M.D.

Boston University School of Medicine
71 E. Concord St., K5
Boston, MA 02118
(617) 638-4310
Director: Robert F. Meenan, M.D.

University of Connecticut School of Medicine
263 Farmington Ave.
Farmington, CT 06030-1310
(203) 679-3605
Director: Naomi F. Rothfield, M.D.

PACIFIC

Stanford University
100 Welch Rd.
Suite 203
Palo Alto, CA 94304
(415) 723-5906
Director: Halsted R. Holman, M.D.

University of California, San Diego
Department of Medicine, 0945
La Jolla, CA 92093
(619) 558-1291
Director: Dennis A. Carson, M.D.

University of California, San Francisco
P.O. Box 0868
San Francisco, CA 94143-0868
(415) 750-2104
Director: William E. Seaman, M.D.

University of California School of Medicine
10833 LeConte Ave., 47-139 CHS
Los Angeles, CA 90024-1736
(213) 825-7991
Director: Bevra H. Hahn, M.D.

SOUTH

University of Alabama at Birmingham
UAB Station, THT 429A
Birmingham, AL 35294
(205) 934-5306
Director: William J. Koopman, M.D.

University of North Carolina at Chapel Hill
932 FLOB, UNC-CH School of Medicine
Chapel Hill, NC 27514
(919) 966-4191
Director: John B. Winfield, M.D.

Source: National Institute of Arthritis and Musculoskeletal and
Skin Diseases, April 1992.

GLOSSARY

Acetaminophen: A pain-relieving and fever-reducing drug used in many over-the-counter drugs.

Acupuncture: An ancient Chinese healing art that involves inserting very thin needles into certain points along the body to relieve pain and promote healing.

Acute: Begins quickly and is intense or sharp; sharp or severe.

Anemia: A reduction to below normal in the number of red blood cells in the blood. A common symptom of anemia is fatigue.

Ankylosing spondylitis: A type of arthritis that primarily affects the spine and sacroiliac joints. Tendons and ligaments may become inflamed where they attach to the bone. Advanced forms may result in the formation of bony bridges between vertebrae, causing the spine to become rigid.

Antibody: A type of blood protein made by the body in response to a foreign substance (antigen). An antibody binds to an antigen and eliminates it from the body.

Antigen: Any substance the body regards as foreign or potentially dangerous, and that results in the production of an antibody.

Anti-inflammatory drug: A drug, such as aspirin or ibuprofen, that reduces pain, redness, swelling and heat.

Antinuclear antibody (ANA) test: A screening test used for several types of inflammatory conditions, and especially useful in detecting systemic lupus erythematosus. It is positive in at least 99 percent of people with systemic lupus. However, antinuclear antibodies may also be formed in reaction to certain medications, viral infections, liver diseases, various types of arthritis and even aging.

Arthrodesis: Fixing a joint through surgery to relieve pain or give support; fusion.

Arthroscope: A flexible viewing tube about the diameter of a pencil, inserted through a small incision into the joint capsule, that provides a view of the inside of a joint.

Arthroscopic surgery: Surgery done on a joint using an arthroscope.

Articular: Refers to a joint. (More broadly, it means "the place of junction between two discrete objects.")

Atrophy: Decrease in size of a normally developed organ or tissue; wasting.

Autoimmune disease: A disease due to the action of the immune system against itself, occurring because the immune cells can't differentiate between the body's own material ("self") and that which is foreign ("non-self"). It is possible that certain body proteins are so altered by viral infections, by combination with a drug or chemical, or by extensive trauma, that they are no longer recognizable by the body as "self" and therefore are rejected as foreign.

Biological: A laboratory-concocted agent, similar to the body's own biochemicals and administered in the same manner as drugs, that alters the body's immune response.

Bone spur: A bony growth around the joints seen in people with osteoarthritis. Joints may appear to be swollen.

Bursitis: Inflammation of the bursas, small, fluid-filled sacs that cushion and reduce friction where muscles and tendons move over bones or ligaments, such as in the shoulders, hips, knees and elbows.

Carpal tunnel syndrome: A group of symptoms resulting from compression of the medial nerve in the wrist, with pain and burning or tingling numbness in the fingers and hand, sometimes extending to the elbow.

Cartilage: A smooth, resilient tissue that covers the ends of the bones so they don't rub against each other.

Chondroitin sulfate: A product, available in some health-food stores, that contains glycosaminoglycans, major structural components of cartilage and connective tissue. Although this product is popular in Europe, there are no good U.S. studies to show it helps rebuild cartilage.

Chromosome: A structure in the nucleus of every cell containing genetic material that determines the characteristics of the cell.

Chronic: Persisting for a long time.

Clinical ecologist: An allergist with a special interest in environmental influences on health. More commonly known as an **environmental physician**.

Colchicine: A drug used in the treatment of gout, usually effective in terminating an attack of gout; side effects may include gastrointestinal symptoms and low blood pressure.

Collagen vascular disease: An autoimmune disease in which the body's fibrous collagen tissues and the cells lining the inside of blood vessels overgrow, causing organ dysfunction and circulation problems.

Complete blood count (CBC): A diagnostic test that measures blood components, including white blood cells, red blood cells and platelets.

Computerized axial tomographic scan (a CT or CAT scan): A sophisticated x-ray imaging technique that produces thin cross-sectional images of body organs.

Connective tissue: A long-fiber type of body tissue that supports and connects internal organs, forms bones and the walls of blood vessels, attaches muscles to bone, and replaces tissues of other types following injury.

Cortisone (corticosteroid): Potent and effective steroid drug related to the hormone cortisol, produced by the adrenal glands. Steroid drugs quickly reduce swelling and inflammation, but do have possible serious side effects.

Culture: The propagation of microorganisms or living tissue in a special medium conducive to their growth. Fluid withdrawn from a joint might be cultured to see what microorganisms, if any, it contains.

Cyclosporine: A drug used to prevent rejection in organ-transplant patients, used with some success in people with rheumatoid arthritis who haven't responded well to other treatments.

Cyst: An enclosed sac or capsule in the body that contains fluid or a semisolid material. Although harmless, a cyst can become infected.

Deep heat: A treatment that uses tissue-penetrating ultrasound waves to heat up small areas of the body; the only heat treatment that can penetrate beyond the surface layers of the skin to a joint.

Degenerative joint disease: Osteoarthritis.

Discoid lupus: A form of lupus that affects only the skin, causing a rash usually across the face and upper part of the body.

Disease-modifying: Altering, changing or slowing the course of a disease.

Disease-remittive: Altering, changing or slowing the course of a disease.

DMSO (dimethyl sulfoxide): A solvent, unproven to work, that is sometimes applied to swollen, painful joints.

Echocardiogram: A test that uses sound waves to detect fluid around the heart and other heart abnormalities.

Eicosapentaenoic acid (EPA): Omega-3 fatty acids, found in fish such as mackerel, sardines and salmon, and shown to inhibit inflammation in the body.

Environmental physician: A doctor with a special interest in the impact that environment—air, water, food, toxins—has on the health of an individual. These doctors were formerly called clinical ecologists.

Erythrocyte sedimentation rate: A test that measures how fast red blood cells cling together, fall and settle to the bottom of a test tube. The more inflammatory proteins found in the blood, the faster these cells clump together and sink.

Fasting: Abstaining from food.

Fibromyalgia: A disease involving pain in muscles or joints with no clinical signs of inflammation.

Fibrous: Composed of or containing fibers. Ligaments, for instance, are rubbery bands of strong fibrous tissue.

Flare-up: A period of time when symptoms worsen.

Gamma-interferon: A medicinal preparation derived from live cells that is being tried experimentally in the treatment of RA and other rheumatic diseases. A biochemical produced by certain of the body's immune cells, gamma-interferon has a range of effects on the body's immune system.

Gamma-linolenic acid (GLA): A fatty acid, found in high concentrations in black-currant oil, evening-primrose oil and borage oil, and thought to have anti-inflammatory actions in the body.

Genetic markers: Specific genes or groups of genes on chromosomes that indicate a particular genetic tendency, including a tendency to develop certain types of diseases.

Glucose: Sugar.

Glycosaminoglycans: Major structural components of cartilage and connective tissue. Available as chondroitin sulfate.

Gold salts: Gold compounds, given by injection or orally, used in the treatment of rheumatoid arthritis.

Gout: A form of arthritis caused by deposits of uric acid crystals in the joint. Gout usually strikes a single joint, often the big toe and often with sudden, severe pain.

Hematocrit: The volume percentage of red blood cells in whole blood.

Hemoglobin: A protein that transports oxygen in the blood.

Hemorrhage: The escape of blood from a ruptured vessel. Hemorrhage can be external, internal or into the skin or other tissues.

Hydroxychloroquine: An antimalaria drug (brand name Plaquenil) that is used to treat rheumatoid arthritis.

Ibuprofen: A nonsteroid anti-inflmmatory agent.

Immunosuppressive: Inhibiting the immune system in a way that interferes with the formation of antibodies.

Immunotoxin: A monoclonal antibody that contains a toxin. The antibody kills a targeted immune cell and thus represses inflammation.

Infectious arthritis: A type of arthritis caused by an infection somewhere in the body. The infection travels to the joint.

Inflammation: The body's protective response to an injury or infection. The classic signs—heat, redness, swelling and pain—are produced as a result of biochemicals secreted by the body's infection-fighting immune cells as they attempt to wall off and destroy any germs, and to break down and remove damaged tissue.

Joint capsule: A tough, fibrous, fluid-filled tissue that completely surrounds a joint. Synovial cells lining the joint capsule secrete fluid that keeps the joint lubricated.

Juvenile rheumatoid arthritis: Any type of arthritis that develops in children. There are several subtypes.

Ligament: A thick, cordlike fiber that attaches to bones to keep them in correct alignment.

Liver biopsy: A surgical procedure that removes a bit of liver tissue for examination. The tissue is procured using a long, hollow-core needle, which is inserted through the skin into the liver.

Lupus: See systemic lupus erythematosus.

Lyme disease: A type of arthritis caused by bacteria transmitted by a tick that infests a variety of animals, including deer, mice and domestic animals such as dogs.

Lymphoma: Cancer of the lymph glands, which are part of the immune system.

Magnetic resonance imaging (MRI): A noninvasive medical procedure that can produce images of soft tissues that would not be seen on an x-ray.

Mast cell: A type of immune cell, often found on the surface linings of organs, that is involved in allergic reactions.

Methotrexate: A powerful drug, with many potential side effects, used in the treatment of rheumatoid arthritis.

Minocycline: A form of the antibiotic tetracycline currently being tested in a clinical trial as a treatment for rheumatoid arthritis.

Monoclonal antibody: A laboratory-replicated antibody being used experimentally to diminish inflammatory reactions in the body.

Neuritis: Inflammation of nerves.

Nightshade: A botanical family that includes potatoes, eggplants, tomatoes, peppers (red and green bell peppers, chili peppers and paprika) and that some people believe can cause joint inflammation.

Nitrates: Food preservatives found in cured meats and some other foods that may cause joint swelling in some people.

Nonsteroidal anti-inflammatory drugs (NSAIDs): A group of drugs having pain-relieving, fever-reducing and anti-inflammatory effects due to their ability to inhibit the synthesis of prostaglandins. Includes aspirin, ibuprofen and many prescription drugs.

Nutritionist: A person who provides nutritional counseling. Although some nutritionists are well trained and knowledgeable, anyone, regardless of training, can call himself a nutritionist.

Occupational therapist: A health-care professional who provides services designed to restore self-care, work and leisure skills of people who have specific performance incapacities.

Omega-3 fatty acids (also called eicosapentaenoic acid, or EPA): Fatty acids found in fish such as mackerel, sardines and salmon, and shown to inhibit inflammation in the body.

Orthopedist (or orthopedic surgeon): A doctor who specializes in surgery of the joints and related structures.

Oscilloscope: An instrument that displays a visual representation of electrical variations on a fluorescent screen.

Osteoarthritis: Degenerative arthritis, often caused by joint injuries or old age. The most common type of arthritis.

Osteonecrosis: Death of bone cells.

Penicillamine: A drug, related to penicillin, that is sometimes used to treat rheumatoid arthritis.

Pericarditis: Inflammation of the pericardium, the fibrous tissue surrounding the heart.

Placebo: A supposedly inert substance, such as a sugar pill or injection of sterile water, that may be given under the guise of effective treatment. In "controlled" clinical research studies, a group of people taking a placebo is compared with a group receiving the treatment being studied. The placebo group is called the "control group." Studies show that about one-third of the people taking a placebo—for any reason—show an improvement in symptoms, at least initially. That phenomenon is called the "placebo response."

Plaquenil: Brand name for an anti-malaria drug (hydroxy-chloroquine) that is also used to treat rheumatoid arthritis.

Platelet: Disk-shaped blood element that tends to adhere to damaged or uneven surfaces and help blood to clot.

Primary-care physician: The doctor you're most likely to see first for most illnesses. May be a general practitioner, a family practitioner or an internist.

Prostaglandin: Hormonelike substance produced in the body from fatty acids. Prostaglandins have a variety of effects, including the control of inflammation.

Psychologist: A nonmedical professional (usually with a Ph.D. in psychology) who may offer various forms of psychotherapy. A psychologist cannot prescribe drugs.

Purine: Protein compound, found in anchovies, organ meats, mushrooms and other foods, that can aggravate gout by elevating body levels of uric acid, which crystallizes in joints.

Range-of-motion exercise: Exercise specifically designed to keep a joint flexible.

Registered Dietitian (R.D.): A nutritional counselor who has been certified in dietetics by the American Dietetic Association (ADA).

Remission: Diminution or abatement of the symptoms of a disease.

Revision: An operation to repair or replace an artificial joint that has loosened, broken or become infected.

Rheumatic disease: A condition that involves inflammation and degeneration of connective tissues and related structures. Such diseases can affect the joints, muscles, tendons and ligaments, heart and lungs, skin and eyes, as well as the protective coverings of some internal organs.

Rheumatoid arthritis: A chronic disease with inflammatory changes occurring throughout the body's connective tissues.

Rheumatoid factor: A protein, found in the blood of many people with rheumatoid arthritis, that indicates the presence of inflammation in the body.

Rheumatoid nodule: Small round or oval bump just under the skin found in some people with rheumatoid arthritis.

Rheumatologist: A doctor who specializes in the treatment of arthritis, especially rheumatoid arthritis and other inflammatory diseases.

Sacroiliac joint: The tailbone; five fused vertebrae wedged between the bones of the pelvis.

Scleroderma: A condition that involves thickening of the skin and changes in blood vessels and the immune system.

Solanine: A chemical substance found in plants such as tomatoes and potatoes. In large amounts, solanine may produce joint inflammation.

Splint: A rigid or flexible appliance to immobilize or protect inflamed joints.

Sternum: A plate of bones forming the breastbone.

Steroid drug: Potent drug related to the hormone cortisol, produced by the adrenal glands. Steroid drugs quickly reduce swelling and inflammation, but have possible serious side effects.

Subchondral bone: Bone found directly under the cartilage of a joint.

Sulfasalazine: A powerful drug used in the treatment of rheumatoid arthritis. In a preliminary study by Dutch researchers, sulfa-salazine was found to slow joint destruction in people with early RA.

Symmetrical: Equal in size or shape (of the body or parts of the body); very similar in placement about an axis.

Synovectomy: The cutting out of a synovial membrane of a joint.

Synovial fluid: Fluid secreted by the synovium, the cells lining a joint capsule, which lubricates the joint and helps nourish the cartilage.

Synovial membrane: The synovium. The cells lining the inside of the joint capsule, which secrete lubricating fluid. In rheuma-toid arthritis, the synovial membrane overgrows the joint capsule, invades the cartilage, and begins to secrete bio-chemicals that can destroy a joint.

Synovium: The synovial membrane. The cells lining the inside of the joint capsule, which secrete lubricating fluid.

Systemic lupus erythematosus (SLE): A chronic, body-wide inflammatory condition that affects the joints, skin, blood, lungs, cardiovascular and nervous systems, and kidneys.

Tendon: A strong band of tissue that connects muscle to bone.

Tendinitis: Inflammation of a tendon.

Transducer: A device that translates one physical quantity, such as pressure or temperature, to an electrical signal.

***Triptergium wilfordii* (thundervine root):** A Chinese herbal remedy for rheumatoid arthritis currently undergoing clinical trials in China.

Ultrasound: A technique in which deep structures of the body are visualized by recording the reflections (echoes) of ultrasonic waves directed into the tissues.

Uric acid crystal: Tiny, needle-shaped particle that forms in a joint when concentrations of uric acid become high, as in gout.

Vasculitis: Inflammation of blood vessels.

Vegan diet: A vegetarian diet that excludes dairy products and eggs.

SUGGESTED READING

Bucci, Luke R. "Reversal of Osteoarthritis by Nutritional Intervention." *ACA Journal of Chiropractic* 27 (November 1990): 69-72.

> *An interesting review of some of the overseas studies that have been done with glycosaminoglycans in the treatment of osteoarthritis.*

Clement, Carmine D., ed. *Anatomy of the Human Body.* 30th ed. Philadelphia: Lea & Febiger, 1985.

> *If you need to see what a particular joint or muscle looks like, this is the book for you. It's a classic of detailed drawings and available in many college or hospital libraries.*

Childers, Norman, F. *Arthritis—A Diet to Stop It: The Nightshades, Aging and Ill Health.* Gainesville, Fla.: Horticultural Publications, 1986.

> *Details the no-nightshades diet and provides some interesting facts about this family of plants. It also discusses other possible joint-pain-producing foods and food additives.*

Dollwet, Helmar H.A. *The Copper Bracelet and Arthritis.* New York: Vantage Press, 1981.

> *Not really scientific, this book is mostly anecdotal, but it contains chapters on the role of copper in nutrition and a possible scientific basis for the copper bracelet.*

Fischbach, Frances. *A Manual of Laboratory Diagnostic Tests.* 3rd ed. Philadelphia: J.B. Lippincott, 1991.

> *A technical, comprehensive explanation of numerous diagnostic tests.*

Gold, Philip W., M.D. "The Stress Response and the Regulation of Inflammatory Disease." *Annals of Internal Medicine* 117 (November 15, 1992): 854-66.

> *A technical article by leading researchers at the National Institutes of Health that explores theories on the interaction of stress and immune function and the development of inflammatory diseases.*

Germaine, Bernard F., M.D. "Silicone Breast Implants and Rheumatic Disease." *Bulletin on the Rheumatic Diseases* 41 (October 1991): 1-4.
> *A review of the studies and case reports linking silicone with connective-tissue diseases such as systemic sclerosis.*

Hendler, Sheldon Saul, M.D. *The Doctor's Vitamin and Mineral Encyclopedia.* New York: Simon and Schuster, 1990.
> *Along with providing good, practical advice, this carefully objective, readable book examines the claims made for just about every vitamin, mineral, herb and amino acid and other nutritional supplements on the market.*

Hess, Evelyn V., M.D., and Anne-Barbara Mongey, M.D. "Drug-Related Lupus." *Bulletin on the Rheumatic Diseases* 40 (August 1991): 1-7.
> *A review of the drugs that cause lupus and other environmental factors associated with lupuslike symptoms.*

Kelley, William, M.D., et al. *Textbook of Rheumatology.* Philadelphia: W.B. Saunders, 1989.
> *A 2,000 page-plus tome you may not even be able to pick up if you have arthritis in your hands. Details just about every aspect of the treatment of arthritis, from the correct way to evaluate a patient to surgical alternatives and total hip replacement.*

McCarty, Daniel J., M.D. *Arthritis and Allied Conditions: A Textbook of Rheumatology.* 11th ed. Philadelphia: Lea & Febiger, 1989.
> *A good source of technical information on such rheumatic diseases as lupus, scleroderma, sarcoidosis and infectious arthritis.*

Miller, Benjamin, M.D., and Claire Brackman Keane, R.N. *Encyclopedia and Dictionary of Medicine, Nursing and Allied Health.* 4th ed. Philadelphia: W.B. Saunders, 1987.
> *A comprehensive, easy-to-understand dictionary of medical terms.*

Panush, Richard S., M.D., ed. *Rheumatic Disease Clinics of North America: Nutrition and Rheumatic Diseases.* 17 (May 1991). Philadelphia: W.B. Saunders.
> *A special issue of this professional journal provides comprehensive coverage of all current research in this area by experts in the field. Includes fish oils, fasting, "allergic arthritis" and nutritional aspects of juvenile rheumatoid arthritis.*

Panush, Richard S., M.D. "Food-Induced ('Allergic') Arthritis: Inflammatory Arthritis Exacerbated by Milk." *Arthritis and Rheumatism* (February 1986): 220-6.
> *An interesting case report that details the study of a woman with milk-induced arthritis.*

Panush, Richard S., M.D. "Food Induced ('Allergic') Arthritis: Clinical and Serologic Studies." *Journal of Rheumatology* 17 (No. 3, 1990): 291-4.
> *A review of the clinical, immunological and blood tests done on 11 people who believed they had food-induced arthritis.*

Pisetsky, David, M.D. *The Duke University Medical Center Book of Arthritis.* New York: Fawcett Columbine, 1991.
> *This is the abbreviated, reader-friendly version of the textbooks.*

Schumacher, H. Ralph, M.D., ed. *Primer on the Rheumatic Diseases.* 9th ed. Atlanta: The Arthritis Foundation, 1988.
> *Without going into the lengthy detail that a textbook would, this book provides basic details on the diagnosis and treatment of many rheumatic diseases.*

Sheon, Robert P., M.D., et al. *Coping With Arthritis.* New York: McGraw-Hill, 1987.
> *Includes information on the diagnosis and treatment of soft-tissue aches and pains that are frequently lumped together as "rheumatism."*

Sobel, Dava, and Arthur C. Klein. *Arthritis: What Works.* New York: St. Martin's Press, 1989.
> *Based on an in-depth survey of over 1,000 people with arthritis, this book quotes people with arthritis who say what works for them and documents the effectiveness of a host of treatments, both orthodox and outlandish.*

Weil, Andrew, M.D. *Natural Health, Natural Medicine.* Boston: Houghton Mifflin, 1990.
> *A sensible guide to alternative medicine—from sweating and breathing to food and exercise. Includes a section on natural remedies for a variety of ailments, including osteoarthritis, inflammation and rheumatoid arthritis.*

Werbach, Melvyn. *Nutritional Influences on Illness.* Tarzana, Calif.: Third Line Press, 1988.
> *Abstracts and references of hundreds of studies relating to nutrition and illnesses, arranged by illness. Includes rheumatoid arthritis, osteoarthritis and rheumatism.*

INDEX